D1675078

Essentials of Traditional Chinese Pediatrics

Compiled by Cao Jiming
Su Xinming
Cao Junqi
Translated by Jin Huide

FOREIGN LANGUAGES PRESS   BEIJING

First Edition 1990

ISBN 0-8351-2368-5
ISBN 7-119-01186-3

Copyright 1990 by Foreign Languages Press, Beijing, China

Published by Foreign Languages Press
24 Baiwanzhuang Road, Beijing 100037, China

Printed by Beijing Foreign Languages Printing House
19 Chegongzhuang Xilu, Beijing 100044, China

Distributed by China International Book Trading Corporation
21 Chegongzhuang Xilu, Beijing 100044, China
P.O. Box 399, Beijing, China

Printed in the People's Republic of China

Preface

Traditional Chinese pediatrics has made great contributions to the health of Chinese children for thousands of years. *Essentials of Traditional Chinese Pediatrics* systematically expounds the basic knowledge of traditional Chinese pediatrics, and the differentiation of syndromes and treatment of children's diseases. Chinese herbal medicine is the main method of treatment. In order to enhance the therapeutic effects, acupuncture and Chinese massage therapy are also introduced according to actual conditions.

This book is intended for those who are already practising Chinese herbal medicine, acupuncture and Chinese massage therapy and are somewhat familiar with the theory and practice of traditional Chinese medicine. Pediatricians of both Chinese and Western medicine, and acupuncture and massage practitioners will find this book a highly useful reference text.

December 1988
Nanjing College of Traditional
Chinese Medicine

The Compilers

CONTENTS

Part One
Basic Knowledge of Traditional Chinese Pediatrics   1

Chapter I Characteristics of Children's Physiology
   and Pathology   3

1. Physiological Characteristics   3
A. Deficiency of the Zang-Fu organs and the immaturity of the body
   and its functions   3
B. Vitality and rapid growth   5

2. Pathological Characteristics   6
A. Susceptibility to illnesses, which develop and change rapidly   6
B. Quick recovery of health due to cleanness of Zang Qi and rapid
   response to treatment   9

Chapter II General Description of the Four Diagnostic
   Methods   10

1. Inspection   10
A. Observation of the expression and complexion   11
B. Observation of the appearance and body movement   12
C. Observation of the tongue, eye, mouth, nose, ear, and anterior
   and posterior Yin (external genitalia and anus respectively)   13
D. Observation of the skin eruptions   16
E. Observation of the stool and urine   17
F. Observation of the capillary vessel of the index finger   18

2. Auscultation and Olfaction   19
A. The cry   19
B. The breathing   20
C. The coughing   20
D. The speech   20

E. Smells   21

3. Inquiring   21
A. Age   21
B. Present illness   22
C. Personal history   23

4. Palpation   24
A. Feeling the pulse   24
B. Palpation of certain areas of the body   26

Chapter III General Description of Treatment   27

1. Characteristics of Prescribing Herbs for Children   28
A. Treatment stops in the middle stage   28
B. Application of suitable forms of herbs   28
C. Dosage of Chinese herbs for children   29
D. Methods of administration   29

2. Characteristics of Acupuncture and Moxibustion
   Treatment for Children   31
A. Needling at the precise acupuncture points without needle
   retention   31
B. The needling sensation must be obtained   32
C. Mastering the needling techniques of reinforcing the deficiency,
   reducing the excess, clearing heat and eliminating cold   32
D. Commonly used methods of treatment of pediatric diseases   33

3. Commonly Used Methods of External Application of
   Chinese Herbs   38
A. Steaming and washing   38
B. Smearing and painting   38
C. Packing   39
D. Hot compress   39
E. Plaster   40
F. Rubbing and cleaning   40
G. Sneezing   41

4. Other Therapies   41
A. Needling Sifeng (Extra.)   41
B. Incision   41
C. Spinal pinch method   42
D. Cupping   43

Part Two
Treatment of Diseases 45

Chapter I Common Diseases 47

1. Coughing 47
2. Pneumonia 53
3. Asthma 64
4. Thrush 72
5. Vomiting 79
6. Diarrhea 87
7. Gan Syndrome (Malnutrition) 93
8. Convulsion 101
9. Epilepsy 111
10. Intestinal Parasites 116
11. Edema 123
12. Nocturnal Enuresis 132

Chapter II Seasonal Diseases 136

1. The Common Cold 136
2. Measles 142
3. Rubella 151
4. Scarlet Fever 153
5. Chickenpox 160
6. Mumps 163
7. Whooping Cough 167
8. Diphtheria 173
9. Epidemic Encephalitis B 178
10. Infantile Paralysis 185
11. Epidemic Toxic Dysentery 190
12. Summer Fever 195

Chapter III Neonatal Diseases   201

1. Jaundice of Newborns   201

2. Erysipelas   201

3. Tetanus Neonatorum   208

4. Disorders of the Umbilical Region   211

5. Sclerema Neonatorum   215

Appendix: Chinese Massage Therapy for
Children   223

Index of the Selected Recipes and Patent
Medicines   227

Part One
Basic Knowledge of Traditional Chinese Pediatrics

Chapter I
Characteristics of Children's Physiology and Pathology

Children grow and develop constantly, while their various tissues and organs as well as functional activities are in an immature state. Despite the fact that along with the increase of their age they are becoming more and more mature, there is a difference between children and adults in the functional activities of the body and its relation to physiological and pathological changes. The younger the children are, the more pronounced the difference will be. It is wrong to regard a child simply as a smaller version of an adult.

1. Physiological Characteristics

A. Deficiency of the Zang-Fu organs and the immaturity of the body and its functions.

This can be generalized as "soft body build, insufficient Qi (vital energy) and Xue (blood), unformed tendons and blood vessels, unevolved spirit, immature essential Qi of the internal organs, and weak body resistance." Therefore, improper nursing will easily cause disease.

Although all five Zang and six Fu organs of children

are delicate, their lung, spleen and kidney are particularly vulnerable.

(1) The strength of lung Qi relies to a large extent on the strength of spleen Qi. Vigorous functioning of the spleen and stomach ensures the strength of the lung and body resistance. Since the spleen and stomach of children are weak, lung Qi and body resistance must be weak as well. This leads to the saying: "A child's lung is often insufficient."

(2) Normal functioning of the spleen implies sufficient source of Qi and blood, rich muscles and vigorous growth of the body. Since children demand large amounts of nutrient substance for constant growth and development, and the function of their spleen and stomach is still weak, relatively speaking, a child's spleen is often insufficient.

(3) Due to the fact that the growth and development of children and their resistance to disease as well as normal functioning of the bone, marrow, hair, ear and teeth are closely related to the function of the kidney on the one hand, and kidney Qi of children is weak on the other, there goes the saying, "A child's kidney is often insuffficient."

Explained with the theory of Yin-Yang, the above physiological characteristic of young children is generalized as "Yang is insufficient, while Yin is not fully produced," or as "the disposition of immature Yin and immature Yang." Here, Yin is used to refer to body materials such as essence, blood and body fluid, while Yang represents various functional activities of the internal organs. The theory "immature Yin and Yang" fully shows that both the material base and physiological functions of children are in an incomplete and imperfect state.

B. Vitality and rapid growth.

Young children grow rapidly in a condition of appropriate feeding like tender sprouts from the earth. They possess the capacity of developing their body build and functional activities vigorously. The younger children are, the stronger and more rapid their growth and development will be. For example, a one-year old baby is 2.5 times as tall as a newborn, while a two-year old child is only 2.7 times as tall as a newborn. A one-year old baby is 3 times heavier than a newborn, while a two-year old child is less than 4 times as heavy as a newborn. Growth and development slow down with the increase of the age. There is also a rapid development of a baby's activities such as turning on the bed, sitting, crawling, standing and walking. A baby is able to learn to do these activities at the age of one. All this explains the vigorous and rapid growth and development of children.

Since children are full of vitality and develop rapidly, they are referred to as having a "pure Yang" disposition by ancient Chinese medical scholars in the book *Classic on Fontanel*, in which reads, "It is asserted that babies under three years of age are of pure Yang disposition." However, pure Yang does not mean absence of Yin, because Yin and Yang depend upon each other. Yang Qi, which is the motive force of growth and development, will have no base if there is no material which is related to Yin.

To conclude, children grow and develop vigorously, despite their disposition of immature Yin and Yang.

2. Pathological Characteristics

A. Susceptibility to illnesses, which develop and change rapidly.

This is because of deficiency of the Zang-Fu organs and the immaturity of the body and its functions. The younger children are, the more pronounced this characteristic will be. As one of the medical classics describes, "The nature of children's diseases is liable to change from deficiency to excess and from cold to heat, and vice versa." This change is more rapid in children than in adults. Children usually suffer from spleen and lung disorders, and also seasonal disorders. Once a disease occurs it develops and changes rapidly.

(1) *Disorders of the spleen and stomach.*

The stomach receives and digests food, while the spleen dominates the transformation and transportation of food, and distributes food essence to various parts of the body. Both of them play an important role in forming Qi and blood and maintaining vital activities of the body. The functions of the spleen and stomach of children are weak, but large amounts of food essence are demanded for rapid development of the body. Improper feeding or inappropriate clothing may easily injure the stomach or induce invasion by external pathogenic factors, thus impairing the functions of the spleen and stomach in transportation and transformation with the ensuing disorders of the digestive tract such as retention of food, vomiting, diarrhea, malnutrition and anorexia.

Due to immature Yin and Yang of children's disposition, transformation of disease easily takes place. For example, infantile diarrhea at the early stage often presents a heat syndrome of the excess type due to retention of damp-heat in the intestines and stomach. When body fluid is consumed, this syndrome will be transformed into injury of Yin. Conversely, a syndrome of injury of Yang will appear in the case of restriction of spleen Yang by damp or prolonged diarrhea due to deficiency of the spleen. Due to the interdependence of Yin and Yang, such critical syndromes as injury of both Yin and Yang may also take place.

(2) *Disorders of the lung system.*

Located in the thoracic cavity, the lung connects with the throat, takes charge of respiration, dominates Qi of the entire body and rules the skin and body hair. When the lung functions well, its Qi disperses and descends. Since a child's lung is insufficient and his body resistance is weak, external pathogenic factors are likely to invade, and thereby impair the lung's function in dispersing and descending, resulting in disorders such as common cold, coughing, asthma and pheumonia. Once a disease occurs, it develops and changes rapidly from a syndrome of the excess type to a syndrome of the deficiency type. For example, infantile pneumonia, especially in severe cases, may rapidly transform from an excess syndrome into a deficiency one or into a syndrome of deficiency complicated with excess. The early stage of pneumonia presents a syndrome of the excess type characterized by blockage of lung Qi due to invasion of pathogenic heat, if the body resistance is still strong then. However, blockage of lung Qi will lead to stagnation of heart blood when the disease develops. Consequently, heart Yang, which is responsible for blood circulation, will be injured, and the transformation of the excess condition into a deficiency one will take place. Clinical manifestations then will include lassitude, pale complexion, cold limbs and a feeble pulse. This is not uncommon clinically.

(3) *Seasonal disorders.*

The Yang Qi of the body is the motive force of the vital activities in the normal physiological state. It is also the main force of resisting disease when it occurs. Children with immature Yang are therefore easily invaded by external pathogenic factors via the mouth, nose and skin, and the invading pathogenic factors are rapidly transmitted inward from the body surface. Subsequently, there will occur diseases with skin eruptions such as measles, rubella, roseola infantum, scarlet fever and chickenpox, as well as infectious diseases such as mumps, whooping cough, epidemic encephalitis B, poliomyelitis and diphtheria.

Invasion by external pathogenic factors may easily lead to transformation of cold into heat, and of heat into fire, thus developing an excess and tense syndrome manifesting as high fever, convulsion and coma. If the body resistance is weak, a deficiency and flaccid syndrome may follow with the symptoms of pale complexion, indifference, cold limbs, and a feeble and thready pulse.

In addition, convulsion is likely to occur when children suffer from seasonal disorders. For example, common cold, a mild illness resulting from invasion of the body surface by pathogenic factors, causes convulsion if high fever is present. Another example is an acute febrile disease, which often produces spasm of the limbs due to extreme heat stirring wind. The pathogenesis of liver wind stirring in children is referred to as "a child's liver is often hyperactive."

B. Quick recovery of health due to cleanness of Zang Qi and rapid response to treatment.

It is true that children's diseases develop and change rapidly. However, the pure Yang disposition of children allows rapid and vigorous growth and development, with a strong ability of recovery. Moreover, etiological factors of children's diseases are often simple, and drastic emotional changes seldom become a cause of these diseases. Thus, a combination of several diseases is rarely seen. Children also respond to medication efficiently. As a result, a mild illness of children can be resolved very easily, and a more rapid recovery from a severe disease is also expected in children than adults if timely treatment is accompanied by proper nursing. According to *Jingyue's Complete Works* in A.D. 1624, "Children with clean Zang Qi respond to treatment efficiently. One dose of medicine will cure the disease if its underlying cause is recognized."

Chapter II
General Description of the Four Diagnostic Methods

There is a common point between children and adults in diagnostic methods. The four methods of inspection, auscultation and olfaction, inquiring, and palpation are applied to both of them. Then the clinical data obtained through these methods are further analyzed. Due to physiological and pathological characteristics of children, however, there is also a difference between them. Babies don't speak, nor can they make their complaints known. Even older children cannot describe their pathological conditions accurately. All this creates difficulty in obtaining information directly from them. Babies are usually not cooperative in the clinic. They may cry all the time, thus affecting their pulse and breathing. As the main approach of the four diagnostic methods, inspection should be carried out during the whole process of the examination.

1. Inspection

Inspection is a method of diagnosis in which examination is made by observation with the eye. It is held in Traditional Chinese Medicine (TCM) that the exterior part of the body has a close relation to the Zang-Fu organs inside the body. Since the muscles and skin of children are tender, and respond to any stimulation keenly, disorders of the Zang-Fu organs are always manifested on the body surface. This makes it possible to obtain clinical data systemically and locally by inspection.

A. Observation of the expression and complexion.

Generally speaking, if a child is active and has a strong spirit with bright eyes and rosy complexion, he is healthy or any disease is then mild. Conversely, if a child is tired or restless with expressionless eyes, he has fallen ill or the disease is serious.

Pale complexion often suggests cold syndromes and syndromes of the deficiency type. Pale complexion accompanied by a puffy face is due to deficiency of Yang leading to overflow of water. This is seen as Yin edema. Sudden occurrence of greyish-pale complexion with cold limbs and sweating indicates abrupt collapse of Yang Qi, seen in prostration. Pale complexion and lips imply deficiency of blood. Pale complexion with perspiration suggests weakness of lung Qi and body resistance. Some healthy children also have pale complexion, which is often tinged with rosy colour.

Red complexion often suggests heat syndromes. Cinnabar complexion indicates wind-heat complicated with toxins, or is seen in scarlet fever. Malar flush in the afternoon implies internal heat due to deficiency of Yin or injury of Yin in a prolonged illness. Light-red complexion of a newborn will subside in 1-2 days.

Yellow complexion often suggests weak body constitution or retention of damp. Yellow complexion accompanied by emaciation and a swollen and enlarged abdomen indicates deficiency of the spleen and stomach, which is seen in infantile malnutrition. Yellow and lustreless complexion accompanied by white patches on the face implies intestinal parasites. Yellow complexion and sclera are the signs of jaundice.

Blue-purple complexion often suggests cold, pain, stagnation of blood and convulsion. Blue-pale complexion accompanied by furrowed brown indicates abdominal pain due to internal cold. Blue-grey complexion is present in mental cloudiness and convulsions. Blue complexion with purple lips and shortness of breath suggests stagnation of Qi and blood due to blockage of lung Qi.

B. Observation of the appearance and body movement.

Observation of the appearance includes looking at the head, hair, chest, trunk, limbs and nails. A Chinese child normally has strong muscles and bones, black and lustrous hair and active motion. Conversely, weak and thin muscles, soft bones, dry skin, withered and yellowish hair, the fontanel failing to close, and dull expression, are all pathological signs. For example, sparse hair, the fontanel failing to close, curved lower limbs, protruding chest, and curved and deformed spinal column suggest chicken breast and tortoise back, seen in infantile weak syndromes. Weak and thin body, and big belly with exposed blue veins are due to infantile malnutrition or to parasites. Withered and yellowish hair or sparse hair which easily falls out implies extreme deficiency of Qi and blood. Purple nails or clubbed fingers result from stagnation of Qi and blood due to deficiency of heart Yang.

A normal child is free in motion and does not show any suffering. If a child likes sleeping on the abdomen, this is often due to retention of milk or food, or to intestinal parasites. Sleeping on the back motionless indicates a prolonged or serious illness. Holding the belly with both hands while shouting, suggests acute abdominal pain. Neck rigidity and contracture of the four limbs are signs of infantile convulsions.

C. Observation of the tongue, eye, mouth, nose, ear, and anterior and posterior Yin (external genitalia and anus respectively).

Since the tongue is the mirror of the heart, the liver opens into the eye, the lung into the nose, the spleen into the mouth, and the kidney into the ear, there is a close relation between them. Disorders of internal organs often take their reflexion on these sense organs. This is an important part of pediatric diagnosis.

(1) *Observation of the tongue.*

This includes looking at tongue body and coating. The normal tongue of a child is light-red in colour, free in motion, and moist. A milky-white tongue coating in a nursing infant is normal.

A pale tongue indicates deficiency of Qi and blood, which is seen in anemia. A deep-red tongue indicates invasion of the Ying (nutrient) and Xue (blood) systems by pathogenic heat, which is present in severe cases of acute febrile diseases. A purple tongue indicates stagnation of Qi and blood, which is seen in anoxia. A thorny and red tongue like a red bayberry indicates toxic heat in the Xue system with exhaustion of Yin fluid. It is also present in scarlet fever.

A thin and white tongue coating indicates invasion of

13

the body surface by external pathogenic factors. A white and sticky tongue coating indicates retention of cold and damp in the interior of the body. A yellow and sticky tongue coating indicates retention of damp-heat or turbid damp in the middle Jiao. A yellow, dirty and sticky tongue coating indicates retention of milk or food. A dry and peeled tongue coating indicates consumption of body fluid and deficiency of kidney Yin. A geographic tongue which appears and disappears from time to time indicates weakness of the spleen and stomach, often seen in dyspepsia. A coloured tongue coating due to intake of certain food, candy, or drugs is not pathological.

(2) *Observation of the eye.*

Attention is paid to the expression first. A healthy child has round and black eyes with a sparkle. Conversely, expressionless eyes or closed eyes are pathological.

Red sclera is due to exposure to wind-heat. Watering eyes are an early sign of measles or a sign of severe common cold. Yellow sclera indicates jaundice due to accumulation of damp-heat in the interior, which is seen in hepatitis. Black spots of sesame seed size in the sclera indicate intestinal parasites. Dilated or shrunk pupils are due to exhaustion of kidney Qi. Slight corneal opacity is a sign of malnutrition. Dull expression with fixed eyes indicates infantile convulsion.

(3) *Observation of the nose.*

Nasal obstruction with watery discharge indicates common cold due to wind-cold; that with thick discharge is due to wind-heat. Long-standing thick nasal discharge indicates retention of heat in the Lung Channel. Ala nasi trembling indicates blockage of lung Qi, which is often seen in severe cases of pneumonia. A dry and irritated nose indicates dryness and heat in the Lung Channel or exposure to pathogenic dryness. Epistaxis is due to accumulation of heat in the Lung Channel, which causes reckless blood movement.

(4) *Observation of the mouth.*

Red and swollen gums with erosion indicate upward disturbance of stomach fire. Since the teeth belong to the bone, failure of the teeth to grow on time is due to deficiency of kidney Qi.

The throat is the gate of the lung and stomach. An inflamed throat indicates invasion by wind-heat. An inflamed throat with swollen tonsils indicates retention of heat in the lung and stomach. A greyish-white false membrane over the throat wall, which is difficult to clean, indicates diphtheria. If the false membrane is yellowish-white in colour and easy to clean, it is a sign of tonsillitis.

Ulcers and erosion of the mouth and tongue are due to accumulated heat in the heart and spleen. White granules on the membrane of the mouth and tongue, which regrow as soon as cleaned, indicate thrush.

(5) *Observation of the ear and anterior and posterior Yin.*

Swelling and pain in the auditory duct with purulent discharge indicate upward disturbance of wind-fire of the liver and gall bladder. Diffused swelling around the ear lobe is due to invasion of the Gall Bladder Channel by pathogenic wind and heat toxins, as is seen in mumps.

Anterior Yin refers to the external genitalia and urethral orifice. A flaccid scrotum is due to deficiency of kidney Qi. Enlargement and drooping of the scrotum on one side indicates hernia, which is due to deficiency of Qi of the middle Jiao. Red and moist anterior Yin in girls indicates damp-heat in the lower Jiao. Itching of the anterior Yin is often caused by pinworms and trichomonas in the vagina.

Posterior Yin refers to the anus. Dampness and itching in the anus with white and thready worms crawling out from the anus at night are due to pinworms. Redness, dampness and itching in the anus and buttocks with greasy fluid oozing indicate diaper dermatitis.

D. Observation of the skin eruptions.
(1) *Fine skin eruptions.*
Skin eruptions as fine as sesame seeds are present in measles, rubella, roseola infantum and scarlet fever.
(2) *Raised skin eruptions.*
Raised skin eruptions, scarlet in colour at the root, often occur on the head, face and four limbs in smallpox, chickenpox and impetigo. Smallpox has been eradicated in China. Chickenpox appears as fine papules first, which then are raised, forming blisters of soy bean size with transparent fluid in the centre and scarlet circle at the root. Then the eruptions dry up and crust. Raised eruptions in chickenpox may involve the entire body, rising here and subsiding there. Skin eruptions of impetigo are turbid with pus in the centre, and red at the root. The oozing of pus may create new pustules around the lesion.
(3) *Spotted skin eruptions.*
Spotted skin eruptions appear in patches, bright-red in colour. They are not thorny on palpation nor do they subside in colour on pressure. They are due to excessive heat toxins in the Ying and Xue systems. The skin

eruptions like this are Yang in nature. Indistinct skin eruptions or dark-purple skin eruptions accompanied by pale complexion, cold limbs and a thready pulse are due to Qi not controlling blood and the resultant blood extravasation. The skin eruptions of this type are Yin in nature, indicating serious pathological conditions.

E. Observation of the stool and urine.
(1) *The stool.*
The newborn and nursing infants normally have loose stool with increased frequency. The stool of a normal child is yellow in colour, neither dry nor too moist. A pronounced change of the stool's colour, form and frequency suggests the presence of disease. Dry stool like a sheep's, and missing several days, indicates retention of heat of the excess type in the intestines or deficiency of body fluid due to consumption of Yin in an acute febrile disease. Loose stool mixed with white milky masses or stool yellow in colour with food residues and bad smell like spoilt eggs indicates injury of the stomach and spleen by excessive intake of milk or food. Stool with mucus and blood accompanied by tenesmus during bowel movements suggests dysentery due to accumulation of damp-heat in the intestines. Bloody stool, soy sauce in colour in nursing infants, accompanied by crying from time to time, is a sign of intestinal obstruction and intussusception.

(2) *The urine.*
Normal urine is clear and light-yellow in colour. Scanty and deep-yellow urine in hot summer due to excessive sweating is not pathological. Frequent and painful urination with yellow urine is due to downward movement of damp-heat. Turbid urine as though con-

taining milk is due to dyspepsia resulting from irregular food intake. Deep-red or brown urine suggests hematuria.

F. Observation of the capillary vessel of the index finger.

Observation of the capillary vessel of the index finger is an auxiliary method adopted by ancient medical scholars in China to determine pathological conditions of babies below 2-3 years of age, in place of feeling the pulse. What's observed is the capillary vessel of the radial side of the palmar aspect of the index finger. The first segment of the index finger from the palm is referred to as "wind-gate," the second segment as "Qi-gate" and the third one as "vital-gate."

Normally, the capillary vessel of the index finger of a baby is red tinged with yellow, and indistinct and unexposed in the area distal to the "wind-gate." Any pathological condition may change the visibility and colour of the capillary vessel. The capillary vessel should be looked at in a bright light. The doctor holds the tip of the baby's index finger with the two fingers and then massages the lateral border of the finger gently from "vital-gate" to "wind-gate" with a finger of the other hand. In this way, the capillary vessel is exposed and the observation facilitated.

(1) *The visibility of the capillary vessel determines the exterior or interior syndromes.*

A superficial and exposed capillary vessel indicates exterior syndromes, while a deep and indistinct capillary vessel suggests interior syndromes.

(2) *The colour of the capillary vessel determines cold or heat, and excess or deficiency syndromes.*

A light-red capillary vessel indicates cold syndromes of the deficiency type, or deficiency of Qi and blood. A red capillary vessel indicates heat syndromes of the excess type. A deep-red capillary vessel indicates accumulation of heat. A blue-purple capillary vessel indicates convulsions, painful syndromes and stagnation of blood.

(3) *The condition of the three "gates" determines the severity of a disease.*

A visible capillary vessel on the "wind-gate" suggests a recent and mild illness. If the capillary vessel is seen on both the "wind-gate" and "Qi-gate," pathogenic factors are penetrating deep, and the illness is then severe. A critical condition is suggested if the capillary vessel is exposed on all the three "gates."

Since observation of the capillary vessel is only one of the diagnostic methods, the clinical data obtained by applying other methods must also be analyzed in making differentiation. It is not correct to rely simply on observation of the capillary vessel.

2. Auscultation and Olfaction

Auscultation and olfaction are methods of diagnosis consisting of listening and smelling. Listening includes application of the stethoscope.

A. The cry.

A healthy baby cries in a strong voice with tears. Crying for a long time while sucking fingers, or doing sucking movement, is due to hunger. Shouting in a high-pitched voice from time to time often suggests abdominal pain. Generally, crying in a strong voice

19

indicates an excess condition, while crying in a weak voice suggests a deficiency one.

B. The breathing.

Shortness of breath, asthmatic breathing, ala nasi trembling, and gurgling with sputum in the throat indicate accumulated phlegm blocking the lung. Asthmatic breathing with the shoulders raised, dyspnea, restlessness, hoarse voice, and blue-purple complexion and lips are critical signs of throat obstruction due to a sore throat. Feeble respiration accompanied by weeping-like vocal sound when breathing in suggests collapse of lung Qi due to respiratory failure.

C. The coughing.

Coughing in a coarse voice accompanied by expectorable sputum and nasal obstruction indicates exposure to wind-cold. Coughing in a restrained voice with yellow and thick sputum which is difficult to expectorate suggests retention of heat in the lung. Long-standing coughing in a hoarse voice implies deficiency of lung Yin. Continuous coughing with exacerbated spells and an echoing sound, accompanied by redness of the face and eyes, implies whooping cough. Coughing in a hoarse voice with a sound as of striking broken bamboo indicates laryngitis or diphtheria.

D. The speech.

The speech of a normal child who speaks is clear and loud. Speaking feebly in low tones indicates deficiency of Qi in a severe disease. Shouting in high pitch is often caused by violent pain. Incoherent babbling suggests invasion of the Ying (nutrient) system by fire in an acute febrile disease. A hoarse voice implies disorders of the throat or vocal cords.

E. Smells.
Foul breath accompanied by ulcers in the mouth or gums indicates heat in the stomach. Belching, acid regurgitation and smelly stool are due to excessive intake of milk or food.

3. Inquiring

Inquiring is an important method of collecting children's pathological conditions. The method of applying it to children is almost the same as to adults. Since babies don't speak, the information is mainly obtained from their parents or nurses. Some older children cannot express themselves clearly either. So, inquiries should be made attentively and patiently.

A. Age.
Asking about age is of great significance for diagnosis and treatment. For example, the diagnosis of neonate jaundice and tetanus is related to the number of days after birth. Herbs bitter and cold, or pungent and hot in nature, and herbs with a strong action of eliminating pathogenic factors should be prescribed with caution for babies. It is necessary to ask about the exact date of a baby's birth. The age of newborns is calculated in days, that of nursing infants in months, and that of more-than-one-year-old children in years. By age the standard body weight and physiological development can be inferred, and proper preventive inoculation suggested.

B. Present illness.

Inquiries should be made concerning the history, location and nature of a present illness.

(1) *Chills and fever.*

Babies with chills often lie closely against the breast of the mother with the body curled up. Older children can express complaints. Chills, fever and absence of perspiration indicate invasion by external pathogenic wind-cold. Fever and aversion to wind accompanied by perspiration suggest exposure to wind-heat. Persistent fever and absence of chills imply inward transmission of pathogenic heat. Chills and absence of fever are due to internal cold or deficiency of Yang.

(2) *Perspiration.*

Normally, a baby sweats slightly on the forehead during sleeping. Spontaneous sweating occurs during the day time on slight exertion, indicating deficiency of Qi. Sweating that occurs during sleep and stops upon wakening is known as night sweating. It is usually a sign of deficiency of Yin or deficiency of both Qi and Yin.

(3) *Head and body.*

Older children are able to complain of headache or dizziness. Headache is often present in fever, while dizziness is in anemia. Headache accompanied by fever and chills indicates invasion by external pathogenic wind-cold. Headache with high fever, vomiting, convulsions, and coma is a sign of invasion of the heart and liver by pathogenic factors. Fever in combination of general aching often suggests exposure to external pathogenic factors of rheumatism.

(4) *Diet.*

Poor appetite with fullness and a distending sensation in the abdomen is due to excessive intake of milk or food. Excessive eating and anal discharge with emaciation are caused by hyperfunction of the stomach and hyperfunction of the spleen, seen in infantile malnutrition.

(5) *Chest and abdomen.*

Stabbing pain in the chest accompanied by fever and coughing is due to invasion of the lung by pathogenic heat, which blocks lung Qi. Fullness and a distending sensation in the epigastrium and abdomen are caused by retention of food. Pain around the umbilicus indicates ascariasis. An abrupt occurrence of colicky pain in the right upper abdominal area as though something were drilling upward from time to time, accompanied by perspiration, a cold sensation in the body, and pale complexion, would suggest biliary ascariasis.

(6) *Sleep.*

Restlessness and cries soon after sleeping accompanied by itching in the anus indicate pinworms. If a nursing baby does not sleep at night or cries at midnight for a long time, this is due to insufficient milk feeding.

(7) *Other.*

This includes information related to the disease such as external stimulation (fear and fright), history of contracting infectious disease, treatment taken before, and the result of that treatment.

C. Personal history.

Included is labour, feeding, development, and preventive inoculation. The history of labour consists of the number of pregnancies, the number of labours, premature or mature labour, smooth labour or difficult labour, the method of delivery, the condition upon birth, and nutrient and health conditions of mother during pregnancy. The history of feeding deals with the mode of feeding and the food the baby eats. Eating habit and partiality for a particular kind of food should be asked about if the child has grown older. The history of development includes that of body build and intelligence such as when the child started sitting, standing, walking and speaking. The history of preventive inoculation includes the age the child received various vaccines and the reaction to them. All this should be made clear and written down in case records.

4. Palpation

Palpation is a method of diagnosis in which the pathological conditions are detected by palpating, feeling and pressing certain areas of the body. Here is included feeling the pulse and also palpation of certain areas of the body.

A. Feeling the pulse.

Feeling the pulse for children is more simple than for adults, because the three regions of the pulse, *cun*, *guan* and *chi* are indistinquishable, and the method "application of one finger to determine the conditions of the three regions of the pulse" is adopted for children. A child's pulse is less significant than an adult's. The younger the child is, the more rapid the pulse will be. Nursing and cries may make the pulse even more rapid. Therefore, the pulse must be felt when the child is asleep or quiet in order to get the correct information. There are six main pulses of children, namely, superficial, deep, slow, rapid, forceful, and weak.

The pulse that responds to the finger when pressed lightly is superficial, indicating exterior syndromes. A superficial and forceful pulse indicates exterior syndromes of the excess type, while a superficial and weak pulse indicates exterior syndromes of the deficiency type. The pulse felt only upon heavy pressure is deep, indicating interior syndromes. A deep and forceful pulse indicates interior syndromes of the excess type, while a deep and weak pulse indicates interior syndromes of the deficiency type. The normal speed of children's pulse is as follows:

Newborn: 120-140 beats per minute (7-8 beats per breath of an adult).

One-year-old: 110-120 beats per minute (6-7 beats per breath of an adult).

Four-year-old: 110 beats per minute (6 beats per breath of an adult).

Eight-year-old: 90 beats per minute (5 beats per breath of an adult).

Fourteen-year-old: 75-80 beats per minute.

A slow pulse indicates cold syndrome. A slow and forceful pulse indicates cold syndromes of the excess type, while a slow and weak pulse indicates cold syndromes of the deficiency type. A rapid pulse indicates heat syndromes. A rapid and forceful pulse indicates heat syndromes of the excess type, while a rapid and weak pulse indicates heat syndromes of the deficiency type.

Clinically, the capillary vessel of the index finger of nursing babies is observed to help pulse diagnosis.

The following abnormal pulses are also present in pediatric clinics. A wiry pulse suggests abdominal pain and convulsion. A rolling pulse is due to accumulation of excessive phlegm-heat or to retention of food. A weak floating pulse indicates either deficiency of Qi and blood or an invasion of pathogenic damp.

B. Palpation of certain areas of the body.

Certain areas of the body such as the skin, head and neck, chest and abdomen, and four limbs, are palpated and pressed.

(1) *The skin.*

Cold skin with excessive perspiration indicates deficiency of Yang and Weiqi (defensive Qi). Hot skin without perspiration indicates invasion of the body surface by external pathogenic factors. Swollen skin which shows pitting when pressed indicates edema due to retention of damp. Pitting disappearing when the flesh is released indicates edema due to invasion of the lung by pathogenic wind and impaired function of the lung in regulating the water passage. Dry skin with impaired elasticity indicates dehydration due to consumption of Qi and body fluid.

(2) *The head and neck.*

Normally, babies below 12-18 months of age have slightly concave head, because the fontanel has not yet completely closed. Incomplete closure of the fontanel after this age is due to deficiency of kidney Qi, which fails to produce marrow. Concave fontanel after vomiting and diarrhea is due to lack of body fluid. Raised fontanel accompanied by high fever and vomiting indicates flaring up of fire and heat, and is often present in an acute febrile disease. Painful lymph nodes in the neck accompanied by fever are due to phlegm toxins. Nodules of varying sizes in a cluster in the neck, which are not movable on pressure, are a sign of tuberculosis of lymph nodes.

(3) *The chest and back.*

Protruding sternum is a sign of chicken breast, while raised spinal column, which is not painful on palpation, is a sign of tortoise back.

(4) *The abdomen.*

A child's abdomen should be soft, tender and warm, and not painful or swollen on palpation. Abdominal pain which is alleviated by pressure indicates cold syndromes of the deficiency type, while abdominal pain which is aggravated by pressure suggests syndromes of the excess type.

(5) *The four limbs and other areas of the body.*

Included in the examination are whether or not the four limbs and spinal column are deformed, whether or not the joints are swollen and painful, and whether or not the fingers are clubbed. Long-standing cold limbs indicate deficiency of Yang. Persistent high fever accompanied by cold limbs is due to the concept that "The deeper heat goes inside the body, the colder the limbs will be." Contracture and trembling of the four limbs are signs of infantile convulsions. Weakness and motor impairment of the limbs on one side or both sides are present in infantile paralysis.

Chapter III
General Description of Treatment

The principal methods of treatment for children's diseases are basically the same as those for the diseases of adults. There are, however, specific features in terms of principles governing prescription of herbs, the method of administration, herbal dosage, methods of external treatment, and other therapies.

1. Characteristics of Prescribing Herbs for Children

A. Treatment stops in the middle stage.

Since the body of a child is relatively soft and weak, and responds to medication with more sensitivity than adults, the dosage and contraindication of certain herbs must be given special attention in application. These herbs include those which are extremely pungent and hot, or extremely bitter and cold in nature, and those with a strong action of eliminating pathogenic factors. Once the pathological condition begins to improve, treatment discontinues. It is not advisable to administer those herbs for a long time. The reason is that herbs which are extremely bitter and cold in nature are likely to damage Yang Qi of the body; herbs which are extremely pungent and hot are liable to injure Yin fluid; and herbs with a strong action of eliminating pathogenic factors can impair Qi of the middle Jiao. Care should also be taken not to cause stagnation when tonics are prescribed for weak syndromes. Oral administration of excessive tonics easily produces stagnation, which is harmful to the functions of the spleen and stomach in transportation and transformation.

B. Application of suitable forms of herbs.

Since herbs in the form of decoction are absorbed by the body more quickly and with quicker results, they are widely used clinically. The action of herbs in the form of pills is slow, but it is convenient to preserve and use them. As a result, pills are suitable for long-term administration. Herbs in the form of powder also produce quick results. Since children usually don't cooperate in taking medication, and it takes time to make a good decoction, it is necessary to reform the forms of herbs for pediatric application. The newly designed forms include infusion, tablets, syrup and injection.

C. Dosage of Chinese herbs for children.

The dosage of herbs prescribed for children varies according to their age, individual difference, and pathological conditions, as well as the experience of the doctors. Since treatment discontinues in the middle stage, the duration of treatment is relatively short. Children usually take herbs bit by bit at intervals, thus the waste of prepared herbs is unavoidable. As a result, a relatively large dosage is prescribed for children. The exceptions are herbs pungent and hot, or bitter and cold in nature, and herbs with a strong action of eliminating pathogenic factors, such as Mahuang (Herba Ephedrae), Fuzi (Radix Aconiti Praeparata), Xixin (Herba Asari), Chuanwu (Radix Aconiti), Dahuang (Radix et Rhizoma Rhei) and Mangxiao (Natrii Sulfas). Generally, the following dosage is applied:

The dosage for newborns is 1/6 of that for adults. The dosage for babies is 1/3-1/2 of that for adults. The dosage for young children is 1/2-2/3 of that for adults. The dosage for children of school age is the same as for adults. Here the normal dosage for adults is the implied one.

D. Methods of administration.

(1) *Oral administration*.

Decoction, pills and powder are all taken by mouth. Decoction should be prepared according to the nature and action of herbs. It is not advisable to prepare too much broth. The younger the children are, the smaller the amount of broth that needs to be prepared. Decoction is taken bit by bit at intervals. If the baby refuses, fix the head and hands of the baby, and then pour the medicinal broth onto the root of the tongue with a fine spoon. The baby will then swallow the broth naturally. The nose of the baby should not be pinched, for fear that the broth might flow to the trachea. A small amount of sugar may be added to the bitter broth to change its taste. If an older child refuses, the parents must explain with patience until he accepts. Pills and tablets are ground to powder and then mixed with sugar water for oral administration. This may prevent powder from choking the baby. Infusion and soft extract are mixed with boiling water for oral administration.

(2) *Nasal feeding*.

The method of nasal feeding is adopted in the case of coma or dysphagia. The sterilized tube is gently implanted into the stomach through the nose and esophagus. The prepared medicinal broth is then taken into a syringe and injected into the tube slowly.

(3) *Rectal administration.*

Insert gently the sterilized catheter into the rectum through the anus. The cooled medicinal broth is then taken into a syringe and injected slowly into the rectum. The catheter can also be connected to a dripping bottle in which the medicinal broth is held. This method not only avoids the difficulty in helping children take herbs by mouth, but also gives good therapeutic results in the treatment of fever, pneumonia, and intestinal and renal diseases.

(4) *Injection.*

This includes intramuscular and intravenous injection, and intravenous drip of Chinese herbs. It is a favoured form of prepared Chinese herbs among many doctors.

2. Characteristics of Acupuncture and Moxibustion Treatment for Children

In the treatment of pediatric diseases with acupuncture, it is necessary to have a good command of basic theories of traditional Chinese medicine and of principles governing the diagnosis and treatment of diseases of internal medicine. Attention should be paid to the characteristics of children in physiology and pathology, while analysing actual cases, determining prescription of acupuncture points and performing needling techniques.

A. Needling at the precise acupuncture points without needle retention.

Babies don't cooperate with the doctor during treatment. They often keep crying, shouting, and struggling in order to escape. If the needle is retained in the point, it will get bent or broken. However, the needle can be retained for a certain period of time if some children above five accept the treatment. The doctor should be kind and try to coax the children to keep calm during their treatment. Once the point is located precisely, insert the needle quickly, then pushes it downward to the required depth. When the needling sensation is obtained, manipulate the needle to achieve reinforcing or reducing effects, then withdraw it immediately. All this should be done perfectly disregarding the poor behaviour of the baby. If the point is not punctured deep enough so that the needling sensation is not obtained, satisfactory therapeutic results can not be expected.

B. The needling sensation must be obtained.

Since babies don't speak, they are unable to tell the doctor what they feel during the acupuncture treatment. However, the needling sensation can be felt with experience by the doctor, who knows that the arrival of the needling sensation is the key to the success of treatment. A medical classic says: "A soft and smooth feeling around the needle means absence of the needling sensation, while a heavy and hard-going feeling around the needle implies the arrival of the needling sensation."

It is necessary to distinguish this heavy and hard-going feeling from the stuck needle and entanglement of the muscular fibres due to the hook of the needle tip. The normal needling sensation does not cause the skin around the needle to rotate along with the needle, while the stuck needle or the entanglement of the muscular fibres around the needle causes circular movement of the skin and creates much pain to the baby as soon as manipulation begins, thus making the baby cry even more violently. In the latter condition, the manipulation of the needle should stop at once. And then the needle is lifted beneath the skin and redirected in the case of stuck needle; and the needle with hook should be withdrawn and never used again.

C. Mastering the needling techniques of reinforcing the deficiency, reducing the excess, clearing heat and eliminating cold.

The needling techniques should correspond to the actual condition of the child. Generally, the reinforcing method is adopted for the syndrome of the deficiency type, in which the body resistance is weak; and the reducing method is applied for the syndrome of the excess type, in which the pathogenic factors are hyperactive. Bad after-effects would result if this principle is not observed. In the treatment of heat syndromes, the needle is inserted shallowly and then withdrawn quickly; while in the treatment of cold syndromes, the needle is inserted deep and then retained in the point for a period of time. For example, coma due to invasion of the heart by heat is treated by bleeding with three-edged needle such points as Dazhui (Du 14), Taiyang (Extra.), Shixuan (Extra.), the Jing-Well Points, Quze (P.3) and Weizhong (U.B. 40). This method clears heat, relieves toxins and promotes mental clarity. Another example is the treatment of diseases caused by invasion of the interior of the body by external pathogenic cold or by cold produced due to disharmony of the internal organs with deep needling combined with moxibustion on points Shenque (Ren 8), to which only moxibustion is applied, Guanyuan (Ren 4), and Zusanli (St. 34). This method strengthens Yang of the body and disperses cold.

D. Commonly used methods of treatment of pediatric diseases.

(1) *To eliminate wind and relieve exterior symptoms.*

This method treats all exterior syndromes due to invasion by external pathogenic factors, and acts to clear heat, cause perspiration and relieve exterior symptoms. The points used include Dazhui (Du 14) l, Quchi (L.I. 11) l, and Hegu (L.I. 4) l. Dazhui (Du 14) is the meeting point of the three Yang channels of hand and foot and the Du Channel, thus dominating Yang of the entire body. Hegu (L.I.4) is indicated in absence of sweating due to invasion of the body by external pathogenic cold. Quchi (L.I. 11) clears heat in the treatment of exterior syndromes.

(2) *To check coughing and soothe asthma.*

This method is adopted to treat coughing and asthma due to invasion by external pathogenic factors, and to act to promote the lung's function in dispersing. The points used include Feishu (U.B. 13) l, Fengmen (U.B. 12) IX, Chize (Lu. 5) l and Lieque (Lu. 7) l. In case of asthma, add Dingchuan (Extra.) l and Shanzhong (Ren 17) l. In case of phlegm, add Fenglong (St. 40) l.

Fengmen (U.B. 12) is the passageway of external pathogenic wind. Feishu (U.B.13), the Back-Shu Point of the lung, promotes the lung's function in dispersing and checks coughing. Chize (Lu. 5), the He-Sea Point of the Lung Channel, and Lieque (Lu. 7), the Luo-Connecting Point of the Lung Channel, are combined to aid the promotion of the lung's function and relief of the exterior symptoms. Dingchuan (Extra.) is an empirical-point for soothing asthma. Shanzhong (Ren 17), the Influential Point of Qi, regulates Qi. Fenglong (St. 40) resolves phlegm.

Moxibustion is applied after needling if the disease is cold in nature, while only needling is used if the disease is hot in nature.

(3) To clear heat and relieve toxins.

This method treats coma, high fever and convulsions, and acts to relieve convulsions, refresh the brain, clear heat and promote mental clarity. The points include Renzhong (Du 26) 1, Shixuan (Extra.) 1 or the Jing-Well Points 1, Baihui (Du 20) 1, Laogong (P. 8) 1, and Dazhui (Du 14) 1. In case of persistent convulsions, do Taichong (Liv. 3) through to Yongquan (K.1).

Renzhong (Du 26), the meeting point of the Du and Yangming channels, refreshes the brain and promotes mental clarity. Baihui (Du 20), the meeting point of all the Yang channels, refreshes the brain. Laogong (P. 8), the Rong-Spring Point of the Pericardium Channel, clears heat in the heart. Taichong (Liv. 3) through to Yongquan (K. 1) nourishes Yin, soothes the liver and eliminates wind. Bleeding Shixuan (Extra.) or the Jing-Well Points clears heat and promotes mental clarity.

(4) To assist digestion and relieve stagnation.

This method treats retention of food, and acts to assist

digestion and relieve stagnation. The points used include Neiguan (P. 6) 1, Zhongwan (Ren 12) 1, Zusanli (St. 36) 1 and Gongsun (Sp. 4) 1.

Gongsun (Sp. 4) and Neiguan (P. 6) are combined to treat epigastric pain and abdominal distension due to dyspepsia. Zhongwan (Ren 12), the Front-Mu Point of the stomach, and Zusanli (St. 36), the He-Sea Point of the Stomach Channel, are combined to pacify the stomach and aid digestion.

(5) *To invigorate the spleen and benefit Qi.*

This method treats diarrhea due to deficiency of the spleen, and acts to invigorate the spleen and check diarrhea. The points selected include Tianshu (St. 25) IX, Qihai (Ren 6) IX, Zusanli (St. 36) 1 and Pishu (U.B. 20)1.

Tianshu (St. 25), the Front-Mu Point of the large intestine, restores the function of the intestines so as to check diarrhea. Qihai (Ren 6) treats borborygmus and diarrhea by regulating Qi. Zusanli (St. 36), the He-Sea Point of the Stomach Channel, is indicated in disorders of the epigastrium and abdomen. This point not only regulates the functions of the spleen and stomach, but also strengthens body resistance.

(6) *To recapture Yang and rescue the collapsing state.*

This method treats prolonged diarrhea, cold limbs and prostration in a serious disease due to separation of Yin and Yang, and acts to recapture Yang and rescue the collapsing state. Indirect moxibustion with salt is applied to Shenque (Ren 8), and that with ginger to Guanyuan (Ren 4). The number of cones used increases until there is a response.

Shenque (Ren 8) is located in the umbilicus, which is regarded as the root of the life, and where the vital Qi of the body accumulates. Guanyuan (Ren 4), the meeting point of the Ren Channel and the three Yin channels of foot, links with kidney Yang. It is from this point that the congenital Qi of the Sanjiao emerges. Moxibustion with big cones recaptures exhausted Yang Qi and relieves prostration.

(7) *To select points according to symptoms and signs.*

Lockjaw: Xiaguan (St. 7) 1, Jiache (St. 6) 1, Tinghui (G.B. 2) 1, Hegu (L.I. 4) 1.

Staring upward: Zanzhu (U.B. 2) 1, Jingming (U.B. 1) 1, Guangming (G.B. 37) 1, Yongquan (K.1) 1.

Clenched fists: Sanjian (L.I. 3) 1, Houxi (S.I. 3) 1.

Frontal headache: Zanzhu (U.B. 2) 1, Yangbai (G.B. 14) 1.

Temporal headache: Taiyang (Extra.) 1, Xuanli (G.B. 6) 1.

Occipital headache: Fengchi (G.B. 20) 1, Fengfu (Du 16).

Mutism: Yamen (Du 15) 1, Lianquan (Ren 23) 1, Tongli (H. 5) 1.

Deafness: Tinghui (G.B. 2) 1, Yifeng (S.J. 17) 1, Hand-Zhongzhu (S.J. 3) 1, Foot-Linqi (G.B. 41) 1.

Weak body constitution: Qihai (Ren 6) TX, Guanyuan (Ren 4) TX, Zusanli (St. 36) TX.

Pain in the wrist: Yanggu (S.I. 5) 1, Yangchi (S.J. 4) 1, Waiguan (S.J. 5) 1, Hegu (L.I. 4) 1.

Pain in the elbow: Tianjing (S.J. 10) 1, Quchi (L.I. 11) 1, Shousanli (L.I. 10) 1.

Pain in the shoulder: Jianyu (L.I. 15) 1, Naoshu (S.I. 10) 1, Jugu (L.I. 16) 1.

Pain in the hip: Femur-Juliao (G.B. 29) 1, Huantiao (G.B. 30) 1, Biguan (St. 31) 1.

Pain in the knee: Liangqiu (St. 34) 1, Dubi (St. 35) 1, Neixiyan (Extra.) 1, Zusanli (St. 36) 1.

Pain in the ankle: Sanyinjiao (Sp. 6) 1, Qiuxu (G.B. 40) 1, Kunlun (U.B. 60) 1.

Pain in the stomach: Neiguan (P. 6) 1, Zhongwan (Ren 12) 1.

Pain in the abdomen: Zusanli (St. 36) 1, Guanyuan (Ren 4) 1, Guilai (St. 29) 1, Sanyinjiao (Sp. 6).

Pain in the hypochondrium: Zhigou (S.J. 6) 1, Yanglingquan (G.B. 34) 1, Aishi Point 1.

Pain in the chest: Shanzhong (Ren 17) 1, Neiguan (P. 6) 1, Aishi Point 1.

The following table shows the symbols in acupuncture treatment.

Symbols	Implication
1	Acupuncture with the even method.
L	Acupuncture with the reducing method.
T	Acupuncture with the reinforcing method.
•	Three-edged needle.
N	Electric needling.
X	Moxibustion using stick form.
△3	Moxibustion with three moxa-cones.
△	Warming needling.
O	Imbedded needling.
O	Cupping.

3. Commonly Used Methods of External Application of Chinese Herbs

This refers to the application of herbs onto the various parts of the body surface. The therapeutic results are achieved through the properties and temperature of herbs applied. The commonly used methods are as follows.

A. Steaming and washing.

The affected part of the body surface is treated with steam generated by boiling medicinal herbs. For example, steam generated by boiling 250-500 g of Yansui (Herba Coriandri) is applied to cause full eruption of measles.

B. Smearing and painting.

Pounded fresh herbal plants or ointment made from medicinal powder is applied onto certain parts of the body surface in the treatment of disorders of internal organs. For example, Xianmaogen (Herba Ranunculi Japonicae, fresh) is cleaned and chopped into pieces, and then mixed with sugar which is 1/10 of the total amount of the herb, and then pounded together. The preparation should be preserved for 1-2 months before being used, otherwise it may cause blisters on the skin. After that, the preparation is placed on a piece of gauze to be attached to the affected area of the body surface. In the case of pneumonia, the preparation is applied to the back close to the focus. Another example is treatment of mumps with either Xianmachixian (Herba Portulacae, fresh), or Xianwulianmei (Herba Cayratiae Japonicae, fresh), or Xianfurongye (Folium Hibiscus

Mutabilis, fresh), or Xiansiguaye (fresh towel gourd leaf), all of which are pounded and applied to the affected parotid region.

C. Packing

Herbs are wrapped up and then applied to the local area of the body surface. For example, 60-90 g of Pixiao (Natrii Sulfas) or 30 g of Dahuangfen (Powder of Radix et Rhizoma Rhei) are wrapped up and tied around the umbilicus in the treatment of retention of food and abdominal distension. A certain amount of pounded garlic is wrapped up and tied on the sole or the umbilicus for chronic diarrhea. Wubeizifen (Powder of Galla Chinensis) mixed with vinegar is wrapped up and placed on the umbilicus in the treatment of night sweating.

D. Hot compress.

This is to warm the body surface with wrapped heated herbs. For example, 3 pieces of scallion stalk, 5 slices of ginger, and 60-90 g of wheat bran are wrapped up while they are hot, and then the abdomen is ironed with the compress for abdominal distending pain due to accumulation of food and internal cold. Heated fresh scallion and salt applied around the umbilicus and lower abdomen is indicated in dysuria.

E. Plaster.

Medicinal powder is placed on certain areas of the body surface and then fixed with plaster. For example, the powder of Dingxiang (Flos Caryophylli) and Rougui (Cortex Cinnamomi) is placed on the umbilicus and then is fixed with plaster in the treatment of chronic diarrhea. Fine medicinal cakes are made of the powder of Yanhusuo (Rhizoma Corydalis), Baijiezi (Semen Sinapis Albae), Gansui (Radix Euphobiae), and Xixin (Herba Asari) mixed with fresh ginger juice. Then a small amount of Flos Caryophylli powder is put into the centre of each cake. The cakes are then placed on the acupuncture points Feishu (U.B. 13), Gaohuangshu (U.B. 43), and Bailao (Extra.) which is located 2 *cun* lateral and 1 *cun* superior to Dazhui (Du 14). This method is adopted on hot summer days in the treatment of asthma.

F. Rubbing and Cleaning.

The medicinal fluid or powder is applied to rub and clean the affected area. For example, the mouth is cleaned with Bing Peng San (Powder of Borneolum Syntheticum and Borax), mild salt soup, or a decoction of Flos Chrysanthemi in the treatment of thrush and mouth ulcers.

G. Sneezing.

The medicinal powder is blown to the nose to cause sneezing. This method is applicable in the treatment of coma due to blockage of wind-phlegm.

4. Other Therapies

A. Needling Sifeng (Extra.).

Sifeng (Extra.) is located on the palmar surface, in the transverse crease of the proximal interphalangeal joints of the index, middle, ring and little fingers. The three Yin channels of hand pass through it. Needling Sifeng

(Extra.) clears heat, relieves restlessness and regulates blood vessels. This method of treatment is indicated in infantile malnutrition and anorexia. The skin around the point should be sterilized first, and then the three-edged or thick filiform needle is used to puncture this point 0.1 inch. See to it that a small amount of sticky, transparent and yellow fluid flows out from the point. Treatment continues with a frequency of once a day or every other day until no fluid is able to ooze or the symptom of restlessness is relieved.

B. Incision.

Incision regulates Qi and blood, and invigorates digestion and absorption. This method is often used to treat malnutrition and asthma. The operation is performed on the thenar eminence of both hands. After routine sterilization, the assistant holds the hand of the baby and presses the area 1 cm away from the operation site. The operator incises the skin and muscle with a 0.4-cm-wide flat-blade scalpel, leaving an incision 0.4 cm wide and 0.4 cm deep. Then squeeze out a redbean-sized yellowish-white oily substance, which is removed immediately with scissors. The wound is then covered by a mercurochrome-soaked cotton ball and wrapped up with gauze (not too tightly). The whole operation does not take more than 5 minutes. It is necessary to press tightly the wound with the thumb for more than 5 minutes after the conclusion of the operation in order to prevent bleeding. The dressing can be removed in five days. Care should be taken to keep the wound away from the contaminated water before the removal of the dressing. The operation scar will disappear gradually in a few days. This method is not applicable to babies suffering from infectious diseases with skin eruptions, or severe edema, or to babies under six months of age.

C. Spinal pinch method.

This method involves pinching the Du and Urinary Bladder channels, and acts to adjust Yin and Yang of the body, remove obstruction of the channels and collaterals, and regulate the functions of the Zang-Fu organs in the treatment of infantile malnutrition, diarrhea and weakness of the spleen and stomach. The baby lies flat on the stomach with the entire back exposed. The operator stands behind the buttocks of the baby with the index fingers of both hands placed on the baby's spinal column, and loose fists on either side of the back. Pinch up the skin and muscle with the index fingers and thumbs. As the hands move upward pinching the skin and muscle, the ridge thus formed moves upward. Go from Changqiang (Du 1) up to Dazhui (Du 14) generally, or even to Fengfu (Du 16) in cases of night blindness, dryness of the eyes, nebula, erosion of the mouth corner, or redness and erosion below the nose. Then, start pinching upward from Changqiang (Du 1) again, and this is repeated five times. While doing the third manoeuvre, lift the ridge a little once every three pinches. Rub Shenshu (U.B. 23) on both sides in a circular motion with the index and middle fingers for 3 minutes after the pinching is over. Treatment is given once a day, and six treatments comprise a course. The second course begins after one day's rest. This method is contraindicated for cases of high fever, convulsion, diseases due to invasion of external pathogenic factors, purpura, or skin infection.

D. Cupping.

This method promotes smooth circulation of Qi and blood, eliminates cold, and relieves pain. Applied are bamboo, pottery or glass cups with smooth, even rims 4-5 cm in diameter. A small amount of ointment is smeared on the areas to be cupped, in order to protect the skin of the children. These areas are decided according to pathological conditions. Cups are usually attached to the skin for 5-10 minutes. This therapeutic method is adopted in the treatment of coughing due to pneumonia, asthmatic breathing, abdominal pain and nocturnal enuresis.

Place the ignited paper or alcohol-soaked cotton ball into the cup, which is quickly put on the selected point. In the treatment of nocturnal enuresis, Shenshu (U.B. 23) and Pangguangshu (U.B. 28) are selected. For pneumonia with its focus being unable to absorb, Feishu (U.B. 13) or the area just above the focus is chosen. To remove the cup, let air into the cup by holding it in the right hand and pressing the skin at the rim of the cup with the left. It would injure the skin if the cup is removed without letting air in.

It is not advisable to apply cupping to babies under six months of age or babies with high fever, convulsion, skin allergy, edema, or hemorrhagic tendency.

Part Two
Treatment of Diseases

Chapter I
Common Diseases

1. Coughing

Coughing is a common disease of children, which occurs in all four seasons, especially in winter and spring. The incidence is high in babies under three years of age. The younger the children are, the more severe the pathological conditions will be. Coughing of children is often caused by invasion of external pathogenic factors, its duration short and its prognosis good.

When lung and defensive Qis are weak, the external pathogenic wind-cold or wind-heat is likely to invade the lung system via the mouth, nose and skin pores, thus impairing the function of the lung in dispersing and descending. Subsequently, coughing will result. Retention of phlegm-damp in the spleen and lung can also cause coughing when induced by invasion of external pathogenic factors.

Differentiation

Of the following three types of coughing, wind-heat is the most common.

a. Wind-cold.

Clinical manifestations: Choking coughing in strong voice with thin and white sputum, nasal obstruction with clear discharge, absence of sweating, possible fever, aversion to cold, or itching of the throat, a thin and white tongue coating, and a superficial or superficial and tense pulse.

Analysis: This syndrome is due to invasion of the lung by external pathogenic wind-cold, which impairs the lung's function in dispersing and descending. Since the lung opens into the nose, nasal obstruction with clear discharge and choking coughing result. The invasion of the body surface by wind-cold does not allow the skin pores to open and close normally, thus giving rise to such symptoms as fever, aversion to cold and absence of sweating.

b. *Wind-heat.*

Clinical manifestations: Coughing in coarse or hoarse voice with sticky, thick and yellow sputum, nasal obstruction with turbid discharge, possibly fever and aversion to wind , redness and soreness of the throat, a red tongue with thin and yellow coating, and a superficial and rapid pulse.

Analysis: This syndrome is due to invasion of the lung by external pathogenic heat. Retention of heat in the lung is the cause of coughing in coarse or hoarse voice. Consumption of the fluid of the lung results in thick and yellow sputum. Since the throat is the gate of the lung and stomach, redness and soreness of the throat is the consequence of invasion of the lung and stomach by wind-heat. A red tongue with thin and yellow coating and a superficial and rapid pulse are both signs of wind-heat.

c. *Phlegm-damp.*

Clinical manifestations: Chronic coughing with thin and white sputum, which is often induced by invasion of external pathogenic factors, gurgling with sputum in the throat, obesity, pale complexion, a pale tongue with white, slippery and sticky coating, and a rolling pulse.

Analysis: This syndrome is due to weakness of the spleen and lung, which allows frequent invasion by external pathogenic wind. This explains lingering cough. Deficiency of spleen Qi results in pale complexion. Dysfunction of the spleen in transportation and transformation produces phlegm-damp, which is stored in the lung after being produced. Therefore, profuse sputum is the distinguishable symptom of this syndrome. A pale tongue with white, slippery and sticky coating, and a rolling pulse, are both signs of phlegm-damp.

Treatment

Chinese herbal medicine:

a. Wind-cold.

Treatment principle: To promote the lung's function in dispersing with pungent and warm herbs.

Recipe: Xing Su San (Powder of Semen Armeniacae Amarum and Folium Perillae).

Prescription:

5 g of Suye (Folium Perillae)

10 g of Xingren (Semen Armeniacae Amarum)

5 g of Qianhu (Radix Peucedani)

5 g of Jiegeng (Radix Platycodi)

5 g of Gancao (Radix Glycyrrhizae)

5 g of Chenpi (Pericarpium Citri Reticulatae)

5 g of Zhiqiao (Fructus Aurantii)

10 g of Fabanxia (Rhizoma Pinelliae, alum treated)

10 g of Fuling (Poria)

Explanation: This prescription relieves exterior symptoms with pungent and warm herbs, promotes the lung's function in dispersing, and resolves phlegm. Suye disperses wind-cold. Xingren , Qianhu, Jiegeng and Gancao promote the lung's function in dispersing, resolve phlegm and check coughing. Chenpi, Zhiqiao, Fabanxia and Fuling regulate Qi, dry out damp and resolve phlegm.

b. Wind-heat.

Treatment principle: To promote the lung's function in descending with pungent and cool herbs.

Recipe: Sang Ju Yin (Decoction of Folium Mori and Flos Chrysanthemi).

Prescription:

10 g of Sangye (Folium Mori)

10 g of Juhua (Flos Chrysanthemi)

5 g of Bohe (Herba Menthae)

10 g of Xingren (Semen Armeniacae Amarum)

5 g of Gancan (Radix Glycyrrhizae)

5 g of Jiegeng (Radix Platycodi)

10 g of Huangqin (Radix Scutellariae)

10 g of Yuxingcao (Herba Houttuyniae)

Explanation: This prescription eliminates wind, clears heat, promotes the lung's functioin in descending, and resolves phlegm. Sangye, Juhua and Bohe promote the lung's function in descending, and disperse wind-heat from the upper Jiao. Xingren, Jiegeng and Gancao resolve phlegm and check coughing. Huangqin and Yuxingcao clear heat from the lung and resolve phlegm.

c. Phlegm-damp.

Treatment principle: To resolve phlegm and dry out damp.

Recipe: Erchen Tang (Decoction of Two Old Drugs), Sanzi Yangqin Tang (Decoction of Three Ingredients for Conducting Perverse Qi Downward and Resolving Phlegm-Damp).

Prescription:

5 g of Chenpi (Pericarpium Citri Reticulatae)

10 g of Fabanxia (Rhizoma Pinelliae, alum treated)

10 g of Fuling (Poria)

5 g of Gancao (Radix Glycyrrhizae)

10 g of Chaolaifuzi (Semen Raphani, fried)

10 g of Zhisuzi (Fructus Perillae, treated)

5 g of Baijiezi (Semen Sinapis Albae)

Explanation: This prescription dries out damp, resolves phlegm and conducts perverse Qi downward. Chaolaifuzi, Suzi and Baijiezi resolve phlegm by conducting perverse Qi downward, and eliminate phlegm by warming the lung. Chenpi, Fabanxia and Fuling are the principal herbs for invigorating the spleen and resolving phlegm-damp. Add 5 g of Mahuang (Herba Ephedrae) and 10 g of Xingren (Semen Armeniacae Amarum) if there exist exterior symptoms of wind-cold.

Acupuncture treatment:

a. Excess syndromes (including wind-cold and wind-heat).

Treatment principle: To promote the lung's function in dispersing and relieve exterior symptoms. Points are mainly selected from the Lung and Urinary Bladder channels, and are needled with the reducing method. Moxibustion is also applied to the points on the back in the case of cold syndromes.

Prescription: Fengmen (U.B. 12) 1, Feishu (U.B. 13) 1, Chize (Lu. 5) 1, Lieque (Lu. 7) 1.

Explanation: Fengmen (U.B. 12), the gateway of pathogenic wind, and Feishu (U.B. 13), the Back-Shu Point of the lung, both act to eliminate wind and promote the lung's function in dispersing. Chize (Lu. 5) and Lieque (Lu. 7) relieve exterior symptoms and check coughing.

Add Dazhui (Du 14), Quchi (L.I. 11) and Hegu (L.I. 4) if there is fever. Add Yingxiang (L.I. 20) and Shangxing (Du 23) in the case of nasal discharge. Add Fenglong (St. 40) for phlegm.

b. Deficiency syndrome (*phlegm-damp*).

Treatment principle: To invigorate the spleen, resolve damp, eliminate phlegm and check coughing. Points are mainly selected from the Urinary Bladder and Stomach channels, and are needled with the even method.

Prescription: Pishu (U.B. 20) T, Feishu (U.B. 13) T, Zusanli (St. 36) T, Fenglong (St. 40) l.

Explanation: Feishu (U.B. 13) promotes the lung's function of dispersing and checks coughing. Pishu (U.B. 20), Zusanli (St. 36) and Fenglong (St. 40) invigorate the spleen and resolve phlegm. Add Neiguan (P. 6) and Shanzhong (Ren 17) for stuffiness in the chest and difficulty in expectorating sputum.

Other therapies:

a. Ear acupuncture.

Points: Lung, Ear-Shenmen, trachea, nose.

Method. These points are needled bilaterally with equal stimulation.

Needles are not retained. Treatment is given every other day. Or rape seeds are implanted on the ear points and renewed every three days.

Add Spleen, Large Intestine and Sympathetic Nerve if there is profuse sputum due to deficiency of the spleen.

b. Tapping with plum-blossom needle.

Points: Fengmen (U.B. 12), Feishu (U.B. 12), the Lung Channel, channels passing through the arm.

Method: Each area is tapped with moderate stimulation for 3-5 minutes until the skin becomes red.

Discussion

Coughing discussed in this section corresponds to acute bronchitis of children. Attention should be paid to the duration of the disease, coughing sound and sputum, in differentiation. Coughing due to invasion by external pathogenic factors is often of short duration, while coughing due to injury of internal organs is of long duration. Choking coughing in strong voice is due to invasion of the lung by wind-cold; coughing in coarse or hoarse voice is due to invasioin of the lung by wind-heat; and fits of dry coughing with shortness of breath is due to retention of phlegm-heat in the lung. Thin and white sputum indicates cold; thick and yellow sputum indicates heat; and large amounts of thin and frothy sputum which can be easily expectorated indicate retention of phlegm and fluid. Babies usually don't spit sputum, and this should not be regarded as absence of sputum. By listening to their coughing and gurgling in the throat, the amount of sputum can be estimated.

Sick children should rest well, refrain from oily food, and take care not to be exposed to cold, especially the chest and back. Proper exercises are necessary in order to strengthen body resistance when the disease is resolved.

2. Pneumonia

Pneumonia is one of the most common diseases of children, babies under two years of age in particular. Its main symptoms and signs include fever, cough, shortness of breath and ala nasi trembling. There is a high incidence in winter and spring when temperature changes drastically, although the disease may occur in all four seasons. The younger the children are, the more severe the pathological conditions will be.

The external causative factors of the disease include wind-cold and wind-heat with wind-heat even more commonly seen. The internal cause is the delicacy of the lung of children, which allows external pathogenic factors to invade the lung easily. Pneumonia may also originate from other diseases such as common cold, measles and whooping cough.

The lung is diseased in pneumonia. Invasion of the lung by pathogenic wind impairs the dispersing function of lung Qi. Retention of phlegm-heat in the lung blocks lung Qi. Weakness of the body resistance allows retention of pathogenic factors. Either weakness of body resistance or hyperactivity of invading pathogenic factors may produce pathological changes of other Zang-Fu organs. For instance, the critical sign of exhaustion of heart Yang may result from stagnation of Qi and blood; and that of liver wind stirring from excess of heat toxins.

Differentiation

a. General syndromes:

1) Invasion of the lung by wind-cold.

Clinical manifestations: Fever, aversion to cold, absence of sweating, coughing, shortness of breath, thin and white sputum, a thin and white or white and sticky tongue coating, and a superficial, tense and rapid pulse.

Analysis: Invasion of the lung by wind-cold via the skin and hair leads to blockage of air passage and upward disturbance of lung Qi. This explains coughing, shortness of breath and thin and white sputum. Invasion of the body surface by wind-cold inhibits defensive Yang, in which condition, Yang Qi is not able to be distributed throughout the body, and the symptoms or aversion to cold, fever and absence of sweating will follow. A thin and white or white and sticky tongue coating, and a superficial, tense and rapid pulse are all the signs of invasion of the lung by wind-cold.

2) Invasion of the lung by wind-heat.

Clinical manifestations: Fever, sweating or slight sweating, thirst, coughing with sticky and yellow sputum, a red tongue with thin and yellow coating, and a superficial, rolling and rapid pulse. In severe cases, there may occur shortness of breath, ala nasi trembling, flushed face, red lips and inflamed throat.

Analysis: This syndrome results from invasion of the lung by wind-cold which turns into heat, or from direct invasion by heat. Thus the function of the lung in descending is impaired, and symptoms of fever and thirst will ensue. Heat condenses body fluid into phlegm, which explains sticky and yellow sputum. Since the throat is the gateway of the lung and stomach, invasion of the lung by wind-heat will give rise to inflamed and sore throat. The combination of phlegm and heat is the cause of coughing and ala nasi trembling. A red tongue with thin and yellow coating, and a superficial, rolling and rapid pulse are both signs of wind-heat.

3) Retention of phlegm-heat in the lung.

Clinical manifestations: High fever, restlessness, irritability, coughing, asthmatic breathing, ala nasi trembling, constipation, a red tongue with yellow and sticky coating, and a rolling and rapid pulse. In severe cases, cyanosis of lips and gurgling with sputum are present.

Analysis: This syndrome is due to blockage of the collateral of the lung with phlegm-heat. Upward movement of phlegm along with perverse Qi is the cause of high fever, coughing, asthmatic breathing and gurgling with sputum. The blockage of air passage by phlegm-heat gives rise to shortness of breath and ala nasi trembling, or even cyanosis of lips. Constipation, a red tongue with yellow coating, and a rolling and rapid pulse are all signs of phlegm-heat.

4) Weakness of body resistance complicated with retention of pathogenic factors.

Clinical manifestations: Low-grade fever, coughing in weak voice, gurgling in the throat, lassitude, shortness of breath, pale complexion, sweating on exertion, cold limbs, poor appetite, loose stool, a pale tongue with white and slippery coating, and a thready pulse.

Analysis: This syndrome is due to a prolonged illness in which lung and spleen Qis are in deficiency. Poor appetite and loose stool are the consequence of deficiency of spleen Qi. Deficiency of the spleen produces phlegm, which blocks air passage and thus results in gurgling in the throat. Deficiency of the lung is the cause of sweating. Deficiency of Qi and blood deprives the body of nourishment and warmth, and this explains pale complexion and cold limbs. A pale tongue with white coating, and a thready pulse are all caused by deficiency of Qi.

b. *Special syndromes.*

1) Liver wind stirring.

Clinical manifestations: High fever, mental cloudiness, restlessness, irritability, delirium, convulsion, staring upward, neck rigidity, a deep-red tongue with yellow and coarse coating, and a wiry and rapid pulse.

Analysis: This syndrome is due to direct invasion of the heart and liver by excessive heat toxins. Invasion of the heart causes mental cloudiness and delirium. Heat-toxins stir liver wind with the ensuing symptoms of convulsion. A deep-red tongue with yellow and coarse coating, and a wiry and rapid pulse are both signs of excess of heat-toxins.

2) Exhaustion of heart Yang.

Clinical manifestations: Pale complexion, restlessness, cyanosis of lips and nails, cold limbs, sweating, rapid enlargement of the liver, a dark-purplish or pale tongue, and a feeble, thready and rapid pulse.

Analysis: This syndrome is due to serious blockage of lung Qi, resulting in stagnation of Qi and blood. The retarded circulation of heart blood causes cyanosis. Since the liver stores blood, stagnation of blood enlarges the liver rapidly. Insufficient nourishment for the heart weakens heart Qi, causing pale complexion and cold limbs. In the case of exhaustion of heart Yang, the heart is unable to dominate blood vessels, resulting in a feeble, thready and rapid pulse or even a fading pulse.

Treatment

Chinese herbal medicine:

A. General syndromes:

1) Invasion of the lung by wind-cold.

Treatment principle: To relieve exterior symptoms with pungent and warm herbs, ease the lung and resolve phlegm.

Recipe: Sanao Tang (Decoction of Three Ingredients for Eliminating Wind-Cold).

Prescription:

5 g of Mahuang (Herba Ephedrae)

10 g of Xingren (Semen Armeniacae Amarum)

5 g of Gancao (Radix Glycyrrhizae)

10 g of Suzi (Fructus Perillae)

10 g of Chaolaifuzi (Semen Raphani, fried)

5 g of Baijiezi (Semen Sinapis Albae)

5 g of Chenpi (Pericarpium Citri Reticulatae)

10 g of Fabanxia (Rhizoma Pinelliae, alum treated)

Explanation: Mahuang promotes the lung's function in dispersing, and soothes asthma. Xingren conducts the perverse Qi downward and checks coughing. Gancao dispels phlegm and checks coughing. Suzi and Chaolaifuzi discharge phlegm by sending perverse Qi downward. Chenpi and Fabanxia resolve phlegm by drying out dampness. Baijiezi resolves cold and phlegm by providing warmth.

2) Invasion of the lung by wind-heat.

Treatment principle: To eliminate wind, clear heat, ease the lung and resolve phlegm.

Recipe: Ma Xing Shi Gan Tang (Decoction of Herba Ephedrae, Semen Armeniacae Amarum, Gypsum Fibrosum and Radix Glycyrrhizae).

Prescription:

5 g of Mahuang (Herba Ephedrae)

10 g of Xingren (Semen Armeniacae Amarum)

20 g of Shigao (Gypsum Fibrosum)

5 g of Gancao (Radix Glycyrrhizae)

10 g of Huangqin (Radix Scutellariae)

10 g of Yuxingcao (Herba Houttuyniae)

Explanation: Mahuang, pungent in nature, and Shigao, cold in nature, are combined to promote the lung's function in dispersing and clear heat. Xingren, bitter in nature, resolves phlegm and sends perverse Qi downward. Gancao dispels phlegm and checks coughing. Huangqin and Yuxingcao clear heat in the lung.

(3) Retention of phlegm-heat in the lung.

Treatment principle: To clear heat, promote the lung's

function in dispersing, expel phlegm and soothe asthma.

Recipe: Ma Xing Shi Gan Tang combined with Tingli Dazao Xiefei Tang (Decoction of Semen Lepidiiseu Descurainiae and Fructus Ziziphi Jujubae for Reducing the Lung).

Prescription:

5 g of Mahuang (Herba Ephedrae)

10 g of Xingren (Semen Armeniacae Amarum)

20 g of Shigao (Gypsum Fibrosum)

5 g of Gancao (Radix Glycyrrhizae)

10 g of Tinglizi (Semen Lepidii seu Descurainiae)

10 g of Huangqin (Redix Scutellariae)

10 g of Dai Ge San (Powder of Indigo Naturalis and Concha Meretricis seu Lyclinae)

10 g of Yuxingcao (Herba Houttuyniae)

Explanation: Ma Xing Shi Gan Tang eases the lung with its pungent and cool property. Tinglizi clears heat in the lung and expels phlegm. Huangqin, Dai Ge San, and Yuxingcao strengthen the effect of clearing heat and resolving phlegm.

(4) Weakness of body resistance complicated with retention of pathogenic factors.

Treatment principle: To benefit Qi, invigorate the spleen, dry out damp and resolve phlegm.

Recipe: Shen Ling Baizhu San (Powder of Radix Ginseng, Poria and Rhizoma Atractylodis Macrocephalae).

Prescription:

10 g of Chaodangshen (Radix Codonopsis Pilosulae, fried)

10 g of Chaobaizhu (Rhizoma Atractylodis Macrocephalae, fried)

10 g of Fuling (Poria)

5 g of Gancao (Radix Glycyrrhizae)

10 g of Chaoyiren (Semen Coicis, fried)

10 g of Shanyao (Rhizoma Dioscoreae)

5 g of Chenpi (Pericarpium Citri Reticulatae)

10 g of Fabanxia (Rhizoma Pinelliae, alum treated)

Explanation: Dangshen and Shanyao benefit Qi and invigorate the spleen. Gancao benefits Qi and tonifies the middle Jiao. Fuling, Chaobaizhu and Chaoyiren invigorate the spleen by dispelling damp through urine. Chenpi and Fabanxia dry out damp and invigorate the spleen.

b. Special syndromes:

1) Liver wind stirring.

Treatment principle: To clear heat in the heart, cool the liver, calm the wind and promote mental resuscitation.

Recipe: Lingjiao Gouteng Tang (Decoction of Cornu Antolopis and Ramulus Uncariae cum Uncis).

Prescription:

1 g of Lingyangjiaofen (Powder of Cornu Antolopis), to be dissolved in water and taken separately

10 g of Gouteng (Ramulus Uncariae cum Uncis)

10 g of Xianshengdi (Rhizoma Rehmanniae, fresh)

10 g of Baishao (Radix Paeoniae Alba)

5 g of Chuanbeimu (Bulbus Fritillariae Cirrhosae)

10 g of Sangbaipi (Cortex Mori Radicis)

5 g of Shichuangpu (Rhizoma Acori Graminei)

Explanation: This prescription clears heat in the heart, promotes mental resuscitation, cools the liver and calms wind. Lingyangjiao and Gouteng soothe the liver and calm wind. Xianshengdi cools blood. Baishao nourishes the liver. Chuanbeimu and Sangbaipi clear heat in the lung and resolve phlegm. Shichuangpu promotes mental resuscitation.

2) Exhaustion of heart Yang.

Treatment principle: To recapture Yang and rescue the collapsing state.

Recipe: Shen Fu Long Mu Jiuni Tang (Decoction of Radix Ginseng, Radix Aconiti Praeparata, Os Draconis and Concha Ostreae for Rescuing the Collapsing State).

Prescription:

10 g of Renshen (Radix Ginseng)

10 g of Shufuzi (Radix Aconiti Praeparata)

5 g of Zhigancao (Radix Glycyrrhizae, treated)

10 g of Chaobaishao (Radix Paeoniae Alba, fried)

20 g of Duanlonggu (Os Draconis, calcined)

20 g of Duanmuli (Concha Ostreae, calcined)

Explanation: This prescription benefits Qi, checks discharge, recaptures Yang and rescues the collapsing state. Ginseng benefits Qi and tonifies the heart. Shufuzi warms Yang and rescues the collapsing state. Baishao and Gancao protect Yin. Longgong and Muli suppress Yang.

Acupuncture treatment:

a. Excess syndromes (including invasion by wind-cold, by wind-heat, and retention of phlegm-heat in the lung).

Treatment principle: To disperse wind-cold for cold syndromes, and to clear heat and resolve phlegm or to clear heat and promote the lung's function in dispersing for heat syndromes. Points from the Urinary Bladder and Lung channels are mainly selected and needled with the reducing method.

Prescription: Fengmen (U.B. 12) 1, Feishu (U.B. 13) 1, Chize (Lu. 5) L, Lieque (Lu. 7) 1, Fenglong (St. 40) L.

Explanation: Fengmen (U.B. 12) eliminates wind. Feishu (U.B. 13) promotes the lung's function in dispersing. Chize (Lu. 5), the son point of the Lung Channel, is reduced for excess syndromes. Lieque (Lu. 7), the Luo-Connecting Point of the Lung Channel, promotes the lung's function in dispersing and relieves exterior symptoms. Fenglong (St. 40) resolves phlegm.

Points according to symptoms and signs:

Fever: Dazhui (Du 14) L, Quchi (L.I. 11) L, Hegu (L.I. 4) L.

Gurgling with sputum: Tiantu (Ren 22) 1, Shanzhong (Ren 17) 1.

Sore throat: Yuji (Lu. 10) L, Shaoshang (Lu. 11) • (bleeding).

Thirst: Lianquan (Ren 23) 1, Zhaohai (K. 6) T.

Asthma: Dingchuan (Extra.) 1.

b. *Deficiency syndromes.*

Treatment principle: To benefit Qi, invigorate the spleen and resolve phlegm. Needling with the reinforcing method is applied.

Prescription: Feishu (U.B. 13) T, Pishu (U.B. 20) T, Taiyuan (Lu. 9) L, Zhongwan (Ren 12) 1, Zusanli (St. 36) T, Fenglong (St. 40) 1.

Explanation: Feishu (U.B. 13) and Pishu (U.B. 20) tonify lung and spleen Qis. Taiyuan (Lu. 9), the mother point of the Lung Channel, is reinforced to check coughing. Zhongwan (Ren 12), Zusanli (St. 36) and Fenglong (St. 40) invigorate the spleen, pacify the stomach and resolve phlegm.

Points according to symptoms and signs:

Low-grade fever: Taodao (Du 13) 1.

Loose stool: Tianshu (St. 25) 1, Qihai (Ren 6) 1.

c. *Special syndromes.*

1) Liver wind stirring.

Treatment principle: To clear heat in the heart, calm wind and promote mental resuscitation. Needling with the reducing method is applied.

Prescription: Renzhong (Du 26) L, Baihui (Du 20) 1. The 12 Jing-Well Points ↓, Shenmen, (H. 7) 1, Dazhui (Du 14) L, Quchi (L.I. 11) L.

Points according to symptoms and signs:

Convulsion: Shousanli (L.I. 10) L, Waiguan (S.J. 5) L, Yanglingquan (G.B. 34) L, Taichong (Liv. 3) through to Yongquan (K. 1) L.

Staring upward: Zanzhu (U.B. 2) 1, Jingming (U.B. 1) 1.

Neck rigidity: Fengfu (Du 16) 1, Tianzhu (U.B. 10) 1.

Explanation: Dazhui (Du 14) and Quchi (L.I. 11) clear heat. Shenmen (H. 7) clears heat in the heart and calms the mind. Renzhong (Du 26), Baihui (Du 20) and the 12 Jing-Well Points clear heat, refresh the brain and promote mental resuscitation.

2) Exhaustion of heart Yang.

Treatment principle: To recapture Yang and rescue the collapsing state. Needling with the reinforcing method is combined with moxibustion.

Prescription: Baihui (Du 20) X, Yintang (Extra.)1, Shenque (Ren 8) △ with salt, Guanyuan (Ren 4) X, Zusanli (St. 36) 1.

Explanation: Baihui (Du 20) and Yintang (Extra.) refresh the brain. Zusanli (St. 36) benefits Qi. Shenque (Ren 8) and Guanyuan (Ren 4) recapture Yang and rescue the collapsing state.

Cupping:

Cupping, for pneumonia of the late stage with persistent rale, is applied to the lower part of the scapula on both sides generally, or just on the side where rale is obviously localized. Local ecchymosis may occur after cupping, but blisters are not to be caused. The cup is attached to the skin for 5-10 minutes each time. Treatment is given once a day, five sessions comprising a course.

Discussion

Due to difference in the degree of invading pathogenic factors and in body constitution of children, there are quite different clinical manifestations of pneumonia. The pathogenic factors are on the body surface in invasion of the lung by wind-cold or wind-heat. The pathogenic factors are in the interior of the body in the case of retention of phlegm-heat in the lung. The syndrome of weakness of body resistance with retention of pathogenic factors is usually of long duration, and weakness of body resistance is more pronounced than retention of pathogenic factors. The syndrome of liver wind stirring is characterized by convulsion, while the syndrome of exhaustion of heart Yang characteristically manifests as prostration.

In the treatment of pneumonia due to wind-cold or wind-heat, it is advisable to cause slight sweating after oral administration of herbal medicine. The sweat should be cleaned with dry towels. Cleaning with cold water or cold compresses with ice bags are prohibited. The room should be kept quiet and clean with proper temperature and humidity. The lying position of the sick baby should be changed now and then. Simple, less salty and easily digestible food is recommended. For babies, liquid or semi-liquid diet is prescribed in order to ensure sufficient water supply.

3. Asthma

Asthma, a common respiratory disease of children, is

characterized by paroxysmal dyspnea, prolonged expiration and gurgling in the throat. The onset usually occurs at night time, and in winter and spring when there is a drastic change of climate. Most cases are between two and five years of age, and typical ones are often above four to five years of age. This disease corresponds to asthmatic bronchitis and bronchial asthma in Western medicine.

The internal causative factors of this disease include retention of excessive turbid phlegm due to deficiency of the lung, spleen and kidney. The external factors are exposure to cold or heat due to sudden change of weather or inappropriate clothing for the environmental temperature, and contact with anaphylactogens such as pollen, down, smoke, fish, shrimp, paint and intestinal parasites. Induced by the external factors, the retained phlegm in the interior of the body blocks air passage and thereby leads to asthmatic attacks. Asthma at the early stage is of the excess type with the lung disease. Prolonged asthma is of the deficiency type in which the spleen and kidney are involved.

Differentiation

Generally, asthma at the acute stage is of the excess type, and that at the remission stage is of the deficiency type, no matter what the causative factor of the disease is.

a. Asthma at the acute stage.

1) Asthma due to cold.

Clinical manifestations: Coughing, asthmatic breathing, gurgling with sputum, nasal obstruction, sneezing, clear nasal discharge, spitting of thin, white and frothy sputum, aversion to cold, absence of sweating and thirst, a white tongue coating, and a superficial and rolling pulse.

Analysis: This syndrome is due to invasion of the lung by wind-cold. The impaired function of lung Qi in dispersing leads to coughing, nasal obstruction, sneezing and clear nasal discharge. The hidden phlegm and perverse Qi combine to cause asthmatic breathing and gurgling with sputum. Thin and white sputum, a white tongue coating, and a superficial and rolling pulse are all signs of cold and phlegm.

2) Asthma due to heat.

Clinical manifestations: Asthmatic breathing, frequent spells of coughing with little sputum first, and sticky and thick or yellow sputum then, possibly fever, inflamed throat, a red tongue tip with yellow or sticky coating, and a rolling and rapid pulse.

Analysis: This syndrome is due to invasion of the lung by wind-heat or by cold which turns into heat. Heat condenses body fluid into phlegm, which blocks air passage and impairs the lung's function in dispersing with the ensuing symptoms of coughing, with thick and yellow sputum, and asthmatic breathing. Thirst, inflamed throat, a red tongue tip with yellow and sticky coating, and a rolling and rapid pulse are all signs of retention of phlegm heat in the interior.

b. Asthma at the remission stage.

1) Deficiency of lung Qi.

Clinical manifestations: Pale complexion, spontaneous sweating, susceptibility to common cold, a pale tongue with thin coating, and a weak pulse.

Analysis: Deficiency of lung Qi means weakness of defensive Yang Qi, which explains spontaneous sweating and susceptibility to common cold. Pale complexion, a pale tongue, and a weak pulse are all signs of deficiency of Qi.

2) Deficiency of spleen Qi.

Clinical manifestations: Pale complexion, emaciation, lassitude, gurgling in the throat, large quantities of thin sputum, poor appetite, irregular bowel movements, a pale tongue with white coating, and a slow and weak pulse.

Analysis: Dysfunction of the spleen in transportation and transformation means insufficient production of Qi and blood, which explains pale complexion, emaciation, lassitude, poor appetite and irregular bowel movements. Deficiency of spleen Qi also allows production of damp and phlegm, which overflows and thereby causes gurgling in the throat and large quantities of thin sputum. A pale tongue with white coating, and a slow and weak pulse are both signs of deficiency of spleen Qi.

Treatment

Biao (symptoms and signs) is treated by eliminating pathogenic factors during the acute stage for the purpose of controlling acute asthmatic attacks. Ben (the underlying cause of the disease) is treated by strengthening body resistance during the remission stage, while phlegm is resolved at the same time.

Chinese herbal medicine:

a. Asthma at the acute stage.

1) Asthma due to cold.

Treatment principle: To warm the lung, resolve phlegm and soothe asthma.

Recipe: Xiaoqinglong Tang (Decoction of Minor Green Dragon).

Prescription:

5 g of Mahuang (Herba Ephedrae)

5 g of Guizhi (Ramulus Cinnamomi)

2 g of Xixin (Herba Asari)

10 g of Fabanxia (Rhizoma Pinelliae, alum treated)

3 g of Ganjiang (Rhizoma Zingiberis)

5 g of Wuweizi (Fructus Schisandrae)

Explanation: This prescription warms the lung, disperses cold, resolves phlegm and soothes asthma. Mahuang and Guizhi relieve exterior symptoms by causing perspiration, promote the lung's function in dispersing and soothe asthma. Xixin, Fabanxia and Ganjiang warm the lung, resolve retained fluid and disperse cold. Wuweizi consolidates the lung and relieves coughing. Huagai San (Powder for Lung Disorders) is applicable if the disease is mild and of short duration.

2) Asthma due to heat.

Treatment principle: To clear heat, resolve phlegm and soothe asthma.

Recipe: Dingchuan Tang (Decoction for Soothing Asthma).

Prescription:

10 g of Sangbaipi (Cortex Mori Radicis)

10 g of Huangqin (Radix Scutellariae)

10 g of Fabanxia (Rhizoma Pinelliae, alum treated)

5 g of Mahuang (Herba Ephedrae)

10 g of Xingren (Semen Armeniacae Amarum)

5 g of Gancao (Radix Glycyrrhizae)

10 g of Suzi (Fructus Perillae)

10 g of Kuandonghua (Flos Farfarae)

Explanation: This prescription promotes the lung's function in dispersing, eliminates wind, and clears phlegm-heat. Mahuang promotes the lung's function in dispersing, and soothes asthma. Xingren, Suzi, Fabanxia and Kuandonghua send perverse Qi downward and resolve phlegm. Gancao dispels phlegm and relieves coughing. Sangbaipi and Huangqin clear heat in the lung and relieve coughing.

b. Asthma at the remission stage.

1) Deficiency of lung Qi.

Treatment principle: To benefit Qi and consolidate body surface.

Recipe: Yupingfeng San (Jade Screen Powder) combined with

Guizhi Tang (Ramulus Cinnamomi Decoction).

Prescription:

10 g of Huangqi (Radix Astragali)

10 g of Chaobaizhu (Rhizoma Atractylosis Macrocephalae, fried)

5 g of Fangfeng (Radix Ledebouriellae)

5 g of Guizhi (Ramulus Cinnamomi)

10 g of Chaobaishao (Radix Paeoniae Alba, fried)

5 g of Gancao (Radix Glycyrrhizae)

2 slices of Shengjiang (Rhizoma Zingiberis Recens)

6 pieces of Dazao (Fructus Ziziphi Jujubae)

Explanation: This prescription benefits lung Qi, strengthens body resistance and body surface, and regulates nutrient and defensive Qis. Huangqi benefits Qi and consolidates body surface. Baizhu invigorates the spleen so as to produce more Qi and blood to defend the body. Fangfeng eliminates wind and acts on body surface, and also aids Huangqi benefit Qi. Guizhi, Baishao and Gancao regulate nutrient and defensive Qis. Shengjiang and Dazao regulate the function of the spleen and stomach.

2) Deficiency of spleen Qi.

Treatment principle: To invigorate the spleen and resolve phlegm.

Recipe: Liujunzi Tang (Decoction of Six Noble Ingredients).

Prescription:

10 g of Chaodangshen (Radix Codonopsis Pilosulae, fried)

10 g of Chaobaizhu (Rhizoma Atractylodis Macrocephalae, fried)

10 g of Fuling (Poria)

5 g of Gancao (Radix Glycyrrhizae)

5 g of Chenpi (Pericarpium Citri Reticulatae)

10 g of Fabanxia (Rhizoma Pinelliae, alum treated)

Explanation: This prescription benefits Qi, invigorates the spleen, dries out damp and resolves phlegm. Dangshen and Gancao benefit Qi and tonify the middle Jiao. Baizhu and Fuling invigorate the spleen and dispel damp through urine. Chenpi and Fabanxia dry out damp and resolve phlegm.

Acupuncture treatment:

Dingchuan (Extra.) 1, Tiantu (Ren 22) 1 and Dashu (U.B. 11) 1 are needled once a day during the acute stage.

Ear acupuncture:

Ear-Asthma, Endocrine and Asthma Point are selected for various types of asthma.

Massage therapy:

Push the chest and abdomen transversely with the emphasis on Huagai (Ren 20) and Shanzhong (Ren 17). Push the back transversely from the top to the bottom with the emphasis on Feishu (U.B. 13), Geshu (U.B. 17) and Mingmen (Du 4). Push the spinal column and its sides from the top to the bottom. Then press Feishu (U.B. 13) and Geshu (U.B. 17). Treatment is given once a day or every two days. Ten treatments comprise a course. This method is recommended in the treatment of asthma at the remission stage.

External application of herbal preparations:

This method is recommended in the treatment of asthma at the remission stage. According to *Medical Book by Master Zhang,* 30 g of Baijiezi (Semen Sinapis Albae), 30 g of Yanhusuo (Rhizoma Corydalis), 15 g of Xixin (Herba Asari) and 15 g of Gansui (Radix Euphorbiae Kansui) are ground into powder, which is made into 6 medicinal cakes with a proper amount of fresh ginger juice. Three g of Shexiangfen (Powder of Moschus) or Dingxiangfen (Powder of Flos Caryophylli) are placed into the centre of these cakes. They are then applied onto Bailao (Extra.) which is 1 *cun* lateral and 2 *cun* above Dazhui (Du 14), Feishu (U.B. 13) and Gaohuang-shu (U.B. 43) on both sides. This is done once every five days in winter and spring, and once every ten days in summer, three times successively. The cakes are retained on these points for two hours each time, or for only 20 minutes, if ionization is introduced. Generally, the local area will become congested or flushed after the removal of the cakes. Blisters may occur in a few patients. Gentian violet is smeared if the blisters are broken.

There is another method of external application: 3 g of Baijiezi (Semen Sinapis Albae), 0.6 g of Xixin (Herba Asari), 1 g of pepper and 1 g of Baifuzi (Rhizoma Typhonii) are all ground into powder, which is applied to Feishu (U.B. 13) after being mixed with ginger juice. The preparation is applied before bed time and removed the next morning. If there is strong reaction in the local area, the preparation can be retained on the point for 1-2 hours. The treatment is given once every day or every two days, seven sessions comprising a course.

Discussion

Asthma at the acute stage is usually of the excess type. Cold and heat must be differentiated then. Asthma due to cold is characterized by clear nasal discharge, thin, white and frothy sputum, and a white tongue coating, while asthma due to heat is marked by dryness of the nose with turbid and yellow discharge, thick and yellowish-white sputum, inflamed throat, a red tongue with thin and yellow coating. Asthma at the remissioin stage is often of the deficiency type. It is necessary to make clear which of the three organs is deficient, the lung, spleen or kidney. Of the three, deficiency of lung Qi is the most common, next is deficiency of spleen Qi, and then is deficiency of kidney Qi.

During the acute stage, the sick child should be kept quiet and calm. The air in the room must be fresh, and simple and less salty food is recommended. During the remission stage, the child should eat better food, be exposed to more sunshine, and do proper exercises to build up health. Care should be taken not to catch cold when weather changes. Such areas as Tiantu (Ren 22), Bailao (Extra.) and Feishu (U.B. 13) should be kept warm all the time.

4. Thrush

Since thrush presents with a snow-white mouth, it is also referred to as snowy mouth. The clinical features of this disease include white granules which cover the entire mouth and tongue like a goose's mouth. Thrush occurs easily in babies whose mouth membrane is thin and tender, especially those with weak body constitution due to a prolonged illness, or those who have received antibiotic treatment over a long period of time, or new-borns. The prognosis is good, although white granules may spread to the nose and throat, and thereby affect respiration and sucking of milk in severe cases.

This disease results from accumulation of heat in the heart and spleen or from upward disturbance of fire of the deficiency type. The former is due to lack of oral hygiene which allows the infection of toxins, while the latter is due to deficiency of kidney Yin following an illness, which does not allow water to control fire.

Differentiation

This disease presents two syndromes, excess type and deficiency type. The excess type is of short duration and due to accumulation of heat in the heart and spleen. The deficiency type is of long duration and due to upward disturbance of fire of the deficiency type.

a. Accumulation of heat in the heart and spleen.

Clinical manifestations: Fever, flushed face, redness of the lips, restlessness, crying, accumulation of white granules in the mouth and on the tongue with scarlet borders, constipation, scanty and deep-red urine, a red tongue, and a rapid pulse.

Analysis: This syndrome is due to retention of heat in the interior or to exposure to external toxins, either of which affects the heart and spleen. Upward disturbance of pathogenic heat or toxins gives rise to accumulation of white granules in the mouth and on the tongue with scarlet borders. Hyperactivity of heart fire leads to flushed face, fever, restlessness and crying. Constipation, yellow urine, a red tongue, and a rapid pulse are all signs of accumulation of heat in the heart and spleen.

b. Upward disturbance of fire of the deficiency type.

Clinical manifestations: White granules scattering in

the mouth and on the tongue without scarlet borders, weak appearance, pale complexion, malar flush, a heat sensation in the palms and soles, low-grade fever, night sweating. a red tongue tip with scanty coating, and a thready and rapid pulse.

Analysis: This syndrome is due to congenital deficiency of kidney Yin. Improper feeding impairs the spleen and thereby deficiency of the spleen and kidney results. This is the cause of weak appearance and pale complexion. In the case of deficiency of the kidney, fire is not able to be controlled, and thus a condition called upward disturbance of fire of the deficiency type results. This explains malar flush, a heat sensation in the palms and soles, and low-grade fever. Night sweating, white granules scattering in the mouth and on the tongue without scarlet borders, a red tongue tip, and a thready and rapid pulse are all signs due to deficiency of Yin producing internal heat.

Treatment

Chinese herbal medicine:

a. Accumulation of heat in the heart and spleen.

Treatment principle: To clear accumulated heat in the heart and spleen.

Recipe: Qingre Xiepi San (Powder for Clearing Heat in the Spleen).

Prescription:

20 g of Shigao (Gypsum Fibrosum)

10 g of Chaoshanzhi (Fructus Gardeniae, fried)

2 g of Huanglian (Rhizoma Coptidis)

10 g of Huangqin (Radix Scutellariae)

10 g of Shengdi (Radix Rehmanniae)

10 g of Fuling (Poria)

2 g of Dengxin (Medulla Junci)

Explanation: This prescription removes heat from the spleen and stomach with Shigao, Shanzhi, Huanglian and Huangqin. Shengdi cools blood and clears heat. Fuling invigorates the spleen and clear heat. Dengxin clears heat from the heart and calms the mind.

b. Upward disturbance of fire of the deficiency type.

Treatment principle: To nourish Yin, suppress Yang and conduct fire downward.

Recipe: Liuwei Dihuang Wan (Pill of Radix Rehmanniae in Six Ingredients).

Prescription:

10 g of Shudi (Radix Rehmanniae Praeparata)

10 g of Shanyurou (Fructus Corni)

10 g of Shanyao (Rhizoma Dioscoreae)

10 g of Fuling (Poria)

10 g of Danpi (Cortex Moutan Radicis)

10 g of Zexie (Rhizoma Alismatis)

0.5 g of Rougui (Cortex Cinnamomi)

Explanation: This prescription nourishes Yin and tonifies the kidney. Shudi nourishes kidney essence. Shanyurou tonifies the liver and kidney. Shanyao tonifies spleen Yin. Fuling invigorates the spleen by dispelling damp through urine. Danpi and Zexie clear kidney fire. Rougui warms and tonifies the spleen and kidney, and conducts fire downward.

Bing Peng San (Powder of Borneolum Sytheticum and Borax) is blown to the mouth three times a day to aid treatment.

Acupuncture treatment:

a. Accumulation of heat in the heart and spleen.

Treatment principle: To clear accumulated heat in the heart and spleen.

Needling with the reducing method is applied.

Prescription: Shaofu (H. 8) 1, Quchi (L.I. 11) L, Neiting (St. 44) L, Lianquan (Ren 23) 1, Zhaohai (K. 6) 1.

Points according to symptoms and signs:

Restlessness and crying: Yintang (Extra.) 1, Anmian (Extra.) 1.

Constipation: Daheng (Sp. 15) 1, Sanyinjiao (Sp. 6) 1.

Yellow urine: Yinlingquan (Sp. 9) 1, Xingjian (Liv. 2) 1.

Explanation: Shaofu (H. 8), Quchi (L.I. 11) and Neiting (St. 44) clear accumulated heat in Shaoyin and Yangming channels. Lianquan (Ren 23) and Zhaohai (K. 6) promote body fluid and clear fire.

b. Upward disturbance of fire of the deficiency type.

Treatment principle: To nourish Yin and clear fire. Needling with the even method is applied.

Prescription: Yinxi (H. 6) 1, Taodao (Du 13) 1, Fuliu (K. 7) 1, Lianquan (Ren 23) 1, Zhaohai (K. 6) 1.

Explanation: Yinxi (H. 6), Taodao (Du 13) and Fuliu (K. 7) nourish Yin, clear fire and check sweating. Lianquan (Ren 23) and Zhaohai (K. 6) produce body fluid and clear fire.

Annex: Mouth Ulcer

As a common disease of the mouth in children, ulcers of varying sizes on the membrane of the mouth result from lack of oral hygiene which causes the infection of external toxins. This disease may occur in people of all ages, but more commonly in young children.

Differentiation

It is necessary to differentiate heat or fire of the excess type or that of the deficiency type. Accumulation of heat in the spleen and stomach is of the excess type, while flaring up of fire due to deficiency of Yin is of the deficiency type.

a. Accumulation of heat in the spleen and stomach.

Clinical manifestations: Yellowish-white fine ulcerative spots of varying sizes, which mat together with bright-red borders in severe cases, on the lips, tongue surface, mouth membrane or gums; pain in the ulcer-affected areas; foul breath; salivation; fever; constipation; deep-yellow urine; a red tongue with yellow coating; and a rapid pulse.

Analysis: The accumulated heat in the heart and spleen disturbs upward, and thereby gives rise to ulceration and pain of the mouth and tongue, restlessness, crying, or possibly fever. Retention of heat in the stomach is the cause of constipation. A red tongue with yellow coating, and a rapid pulse are both signs of internal heat.

b. Flaring up of fire of the deficiency type.

Clinical manifestations: Pinkish, deep and erosive ulceration of long duration, possibly restlessness, malar flush, thirst, a red tongue tip, and a thready and rapid pulse.

Analysis: This syndrome is due to consumption of Yin fluid in a prolonged illness, which implies deficiency of the spleen and kidney. In this condition, water fails to control fire, which disturbs upward and thus causes erosive ulceration.

Treatment

Chinese herbal medicine:

a. Accumulation of heat in the spleen and stomach.

Treatment principle: To relieve constipation and reduce fire.

Recipe: Liangge San (Powder for Cooling the Diaphragm).

Prescription:

10 g of Huangqin (Radix Scutellariae)

10 g of Lianqiao (Fructus Forsythiae)

10 g of Chaoshanzhi (Fructus Gardeniae, fried)

3 g of Bohe (Herba Menthae)

5 g of Gancao (Radix Glycyrrhizae)

10 g of Shengdahuang (Radix et Rhizoma Rhei, raw), to be decocted later

10 g of Mangxiao (Natrii Sulfas), to be dissolved in boiled water and taken separately

10 ml of honey

10 g of Danzhuye (Herba Lophatheri)

Explanation: This prescription clears heat, dispels toxins, relieves constipation, and reduces fire. Huangqin, Lianqiao and Shanzhi clear heat and dispel toxins. Dahuang and Mangxiao relieve constipation and reduce fire. Dazhuye clears heat from the heart and relieves restlessness. Bohe disperses retained fire. Honey and Gancao dispel toxins and ease the middle Jiao.

b. Flaring up of fire of the deficiency type.

Treatment principle: To nourish Yin and subdue fire.

Recipe: Liuwei Dihuang Wan (Pill of Radix Rehmanniae in Six Ingredients).

Prescription:

10 g of Shudi (Radix Rehmanniae Praeparata)

10 g of Shanyurou (Fructus Corni)

10 g of Shanyao (Rhizoma Dioscoreae)

10 g of Fuling (Poria)

10 g of Danpi (Cortex Moutan Radicis)

10 g of Zexie (Rhizoma Alismatis)

Explanation: This prescription nourishes Yin, tonifies the kidney and subdues fire. Shudi nourishes kidney Yin. Shanyurou tonifies the liver and kidney. Shanyao tonifies spleen Yin. Fuling invigorates the spleen by dispelling damp through urination. Danpi clears liver fire. Zexie clears kidney fire.

Oral administration of herbal decoction is usually combined with external application in the treatment of mouth ulcers. Bing Peng San (Powder of Borneolum Syntheticum Borax) is applied to the affected areas if the ulcers have just started or in less severe cases; Xilei San (Powder for Relieving Throat Erosion) is prescribed in severe cases; and Yangyin Shengji San (Powder for Nourishing Yin and Producing Muscles) is chosen in a deficiency condition.

Acupuncture treatment:

Refer to the treatment of thrush.

Discussion

Oral administration of herbal decoction should be aided by external application of medicinal preparations in the treatment of thrush and mouth ulcers. For prophylaxis, the mouth of children and the nipples of the mother should be kept clean. Take care not to injure the mouth membrane of children. It is advisable to feed the children with various types of food such as fresh vegetables.

5. Vomiting

Vomiting may occur in children of different ages, especially in young children and babies, and in all the seasons, summer and autumn in particular. The vomiting discussed in this section includes that caused by cold, heat, retention of food, and fright. Vomiting, as a symptom, may be present in acute infectious febrile diseases or in acute abdomen, which is not discussed here.

Retention of milk or food, accumulation of heat in the stomach, deficiency and coldness in the spleen and stomach, or fear and fright can all cause dysharmony of the spleen and stomach and thereby result in failure of stomach Qi in descending. Upward disturbance of stomach Qi is the direct cause of vomiting.

Differentiation

Attention should be paid to vomitus and the speed of vomiting in differentiation.

a. Vomiting due to retention of food or milk.

Clinical manifestations: Nausea, vomiting with acid smell, belching with foul odor, anorexia, distending pain in the epigastrium and abdomen which is alleviated by vomiting, possibly fever, foul breath, foul flatus, hesitant bowel movements or loose stool with foul smell, a thick and sticky tongue coating, and a rolling and forceful pulse.

Analysis: Retention of food or milk in the middle Jiao impairs the spleen's function in transportation and transformation, and thereby the food or milk there becomes spoilt; and the function of the stomach in receiving food is also impaired, and thus stomach Qi disturbs upward. All this explains vomiting, belching with acid smell, anorexia and foul breath. Fever is due to transformation of retained food into heat. A thick and sticky tongue coating, and a rolling and forceful pulse are signs of retention of food or milk.

b. Vomiting due to heat in the stomach.

Clinical manifestations: Vomiting with acid smell soon after eating, thirst with desire to drink, restlessness, insomnia, a feverish sensation of the body, redness of lips, foul stool or constipation, scanty and yellow urine, a red tongue with yellow coating, and a rolling and rapid pulse.

Analysis: This syndrome has a quick onset, and the retained food transforms into heat and causes stomach Qi to disturb upward. Thus, vomiting with acid smell soon after eating occurs. Retention of heat in the stomach gives rise to thirst with desire to drink. Dysharmony of the stomach is the cause of restlessness and insomnia. Consumption of Yin fluid by stomach heat leads to a feverish sensation of the body, redness of lips, constipation and scanty and yellow urine. A red tongue with yellow coating, and a rolling and rapid pulse are signs of stomach heat.

c. Vomiting due to coldness in the stomach.

Clinical manifestations: Vomiting long after eating with undigested food or clear and thin sputum-like substance which does not smell foul, loose stool, pale complexion and lips, lassitude, cold limbs, preference for warmth, aversion to cold, a pale tongue with white coating, and a deep and slow pulse.

Analysis: This syndrome is due to deficiency and coldness of the spleen and stomach following a prolonged illness. Deficiency of Yang of the middle Jiao is the cause of vomiting long after eating with undigested food or clear and thin sputum-like substance, and loose stool. The other symptoms and signs listed above fall into a cold syndrome of the deficiency type.

d. Vomiting due to fear and fright.

Clinical manifestations: Vomiting with clear fluid, blueish-pale complexion, restlessness, sudden jerking movements of the body during sleep or disturbed sleep, and frequent spells of crying.

Analysis: The spirit of children is weak. Fear and fright may consume heart Qi and thus lead to restlessness, sudden jerking movements of the body during sleep or disturbed sleep, and pale complexion. Fear causes Qi to decline, and fright causes Qi to be deranged. Subsequently, the liver and gall bladder are disturbed with the result of frequent spells of crying. Invasion of the stomach by perverse liver Qi is the cause of vomiting with clear fluid.

Treatment

Chinese herbal medicine:

a. Vomiting due to retention of food or milk.

Treatment principle: To pacify the stomach and relieve stagnation.

Recipe: Baohe Wan (Pill for Protecting Harmony).

Prescription:

10 g of Lianqiao (Fructus Forsythiae)

10 g of Zhishi (Fructus Aurantii Immaturus)

10 g of Binglang (Semen Arecae)

5 g of Chenpi (Pericarpium Citri Reticulatae)

10 g of Chaolaifuzi (Semen Raphani, fried)

10 g of Jiaoshanzha (Fructus Crataegi, burnt)

10 g of Jiaoshenqu (Massa Fermentata Medicinalis, burnt)

10 g of Chaomaiya (Fructus Hordei Germinatus, fried)

Explanation: This prescription aids digestion, relieves stagnation, pacifies the stomach and sends perverse Qi downward. Jiaoshenqu, Jiaoshanzha and Chaomaiya aid digestion and invigorate the spleen in transportation and transformation. Chaolaifuzi circulates Qi and relieves stagnation. Chenpi regulates Qi. Zhishi breaks stagnation of Qi and relieves accumulation. Lianqiao clears heat.

b. Vomiting due to heat in the stomach.

Treatment principle: To clear heat and pacify the stomach.

Recipe: Huo Lian Tang (Decoction of Herba Agastachis and Rhizoma Coptidis).

Prescription:

2 g of Chaohuanglian (Rhizoma Coptidis, fried)

10 g of Huoxiang (Herba Agastachis)

5 g of Houpo (Cortex Magnoliae Officinalis)

10 g of Jiangbanxia (Rhizoma Pineliae, ginger treated)

10 g of Daizheshi (Haematitum)

5 g of Jiangzhuru (Caulis Bambusae in Taenis, ginger treated)

Explanation: This prescription clears heat, pacifies the stomach, sends perverse Qi downward and checks vomiting. Huanglian clears heat in the stomach. Huoxiang pacifies the stomach with its aromatic smell. Houpo resolves turbid damp. Zhuru, Jiangbanxia and Daizheshi pacify the stomach and send perverse Qi downward.

c. Vomiting due to coldness in the stomach.

Treatment principle: To warm the middle Jiao and disperse cold.

Recipe: Ding Yu Lizhong Tang (Decoction of Flos Caryophylli and Fructus Evodiae for Regulating the Middle Jiao).

Prescription:

1 g of Gongdingxiang (Flos Caryophylli)

2 g of Wuyu (Fructus Evodiae)

10 g of Taizishen (Radix Pseudostellariae)

10 g of Chaobaizhu (Rhizoma Atractylodis Macrocephalae, fried)

3 g of Ganjiang (Rhizoma Zingiberis)

5 g of Muxiang (Radix Aucklandiae)

2 g of Sharen (Fructus Amomi)

10 g of Jiangbanxia (Rhizoma Pinelliae, ginger treated)

5 g of Chenpi (Pericarpium Citri Reticulatae)

Explanation: This prescription warms the middle Jiao, disperses cold, sends perverse Qi downward and checks vomiting. Dingxiang warms the stomach and circulates Qi. Wuyu is warm in nature and sends perverse Qi downward. Taizishen invigorates the spleen and benefits Qi. Chaobaizhu dries out damp and invigorates the spleen. Ganjiang warms the middle Jiao and assists Yang. Muxiazng, Sharen, Chenpi and Jiangbanxia regulate Qi and pacify the stomch.

d. Vomiting due to fear and fright.

Treatment principle: To relieve convulsion and check vomiting.

Recipe: Dingtu Wan (Pill for Checking Vomiting)

Prescription:

0.5 g of Zhiquanxie (Scorpio, treated)

2 g of Gongdingxiang (Flos Caryophylli)

10 g of Jiangbanxia (Rhizoma Pinelliae, ginger treated)

10 g of Juhua (Flos Chrysanthemi)

5 g of Tianma (Rhizoma Gastrodiae)

20 g of Cishi (Magnetitum)

Explanation: This prescription relieves convulsion and checks vomiting. Quanxie calms wind and relieves convulsion. Dingxiang and Banxia pacify the stomach and send perverse Qi downward. Juhua and Tianma suppress liver wind. Cishi soothes the heart and calms the mind.

Acupuncture Treatment:

a. *Excess syndromes (including retention of food and*

heat in the stomach).

Treatment principle: To pacify the stomach and relieve stagnation for retention of food; and to clear heat and pacify the stomach for heat in the stomach. Points are mainly selected from the Stomach and Ren channels and needled with the reducing method.

Prescription: Neiguan (P. 6) L, Zhongwan (Ren 12) 1, Zusanli (St, 36) L.

Explanation: Neiguan (P. 6) sends perverse Qi downward and checks vomiting. Zhongwan (Ren 12), the Front-Mu Point of the stomach, and Zusanli (St. 36), the Lower He-Sea Point of the stomach, are combined to pacify the stomach and relieve stagnation.

Points according to symptoms and signs:

Epigastric distension and foul breath: Jianli (Ren 11) 1, Yanglingquan (G.B. 34) L.

Loose stool with foul smell: Tianshu (St. 25) 1, Gongsun (Sp. 4) 1.

Constipation due to heat in the stomach: Quchi (L.I. 11) L, Daheng (Sp. 15) 1, Neiting (St. 44) L.

Restlessness and poor sleep: Yintang (Extra.) 1, Shenmen (H. 7)1.

b. Deficiency syndromes (including coldness in the stomach and fear and fright).

Treatment principle: To warm the middle Jiao and disperse cold for coldness in the stomach; and to relieve convulsion and check vomiting for fear and fright. Points are mainly selected from the Stomach, Liver and Gall Bladder channels and needled with the reinforcing or even method. Moxibustion is used as well in the case of coldness in the stomach.

Prescription: Neiguan (P. 6) 1, Zhongwan (Ren 12) IX, Zusanli (St. 36) IX, Taichong (Liv. 3) 1.

Explanation: Neiguan (P. 6) sends perverse Qi downward and checks vomiting. Zhongwan (Ren 12) and Zusanli (St. 36) pacify the middle Jiao. Taichong (Liv. 3) regulates Qi of the liver and stomach.

Points according to symptoms and signs:

Coldness in the stomach: Liangmen (St. 21) IX, Qihai (Ren 6) IX.

Fear and fright: Yintang (Extra.) 1, Shenmen (H. 7) 1, Yanglingquan (G.B. 34) 1.

Other therapies:

Ear acupuncture.

Points: Stomach, Liver, Sympathetic Nerve, Subcortex, Ear-Shenmen.

Method: Rape seeds are implanted onto these points on both sides.

Massage therapy.

Push Pitu 300-500 times.

Push or rub with a circular motion Banmen 50-200 times.

Discussion

There are many etiological factors of vomiting, but all of them cause vomiting by impairing the function of the stomach in descending and thereby result in upward disturbance of stomach Qi. In the treatment of vomiting in children, the methods of assisting digestion, clearing heat, warming the middle Jiao and nourishing Yin are adopted according to etiological factors. The method of pacifying the stomach and sending perverse Qi downward is also used to help the treatment. Acupuncture is an effective method in dealing with vomiting. Moxibustion is combined in the case of retention of food or coldness in the stomach. Let the sick baby lie on the side so that the vomitus will flow out smoothly instead of choking the baby. Small quantities of Chinese herbal decoction are administered at short intervals. If oral administration causes immediate vomiting, rub the tongue two to three times with ginger slices. This may help the baby swallow the drug without vomiting. Don't feed the baby if vomiting occurs frequently and violently.

6. Diarrhea

Diarrhea is a common digestive disease in children, characterized by increased bowel movements with loose stool or stool like stirred egg soup. It may occur in all four seasons, but more commonly in summer and autumn. The incidence is high in babies under two years of age. The younger the babies are, the higher the incidence and the more severe the pathological conditions will be. The critical conditions such as damage of Yin and damage of Yang are likely to occur. Prolonged diarrhea injures the spleen and stomach with the result of malnutrition.

Irregular food or milk intake or eating food which is difficult to digest damages the spleen and stomach. The undigested food and damp thus formed combine to cause diarrhea. Secondly, exposure to external pathogenic factors, especially wind, cold, summer heat and damp, brings about functional disturbance of the spleen and stomach; subsequently, diarrhea follows. Thirdly, weakeness of the spleen and stomach following an illness implies dysfunction in receiving, digesting, transporting and transforming food. Water and damp thus produced cause diarrhea.

Differentiation

Differentiation of diarrhea of children is based on etiological factors.

a. Retention of food.

Clinical manifestations: Crying before bowel movements due to abdominal distension and pain, which are alleviated after bowel movements, stool like spoilt egg, belching, sour regurgitation, anorexia, a thick and sticky or dirty and sticky tongue coating, and a rolling pulse.

Analysis: This syndrome is due to accumulation of milk or food in the stomach and intestines. The impairment of function of the large intestine in transmission produces damp and heat, and this explains foul stool like spoilt eggs. Retention of food in the middle Jiao does not allow smooth circulation of Qi there, and thereby gives rise to abdominal distension and pain, which are alleviated after bowel movements. Dysfunction of the spleen results in poor appetite. A dirty and sticky tongue coating, and a rolling pulse are both signs of retention of food in the middle Jiao.

b. Damp-heat.

Clinical manifestations: Diarrhea in a sudden burst with deep-yellow, hot and foul stool, flushed anus, anorexia, crying due to abdominal pain, fever, restlessness, thirst, scanty and yellow urine, a red tongue with yellow and sticky coating, and a rapid pulse.

Analysis: This syndrome usually occurs in summer and autumn due to retention of damp-heat in the interior. Excessive heat acting on the large intestine is the cause of diarrhea in a sudden burst with deep-yellow, hot and foul stool, and flushed anus. The combination of damp and heat explains fever, restlessness and thirst. Dysfunction of the spleen in transportation and transformation leads to retarded circulation of Qi there, and thereby results in anorexia and abdominal pain. Excessive discharge of body fluid through the large intestine causes scanty and yellow urine. A red tongue with yellow coating, and a rapid pulse, are all signs of retention of damp heat in the intestines.

c. Deficiency of the spleen.

Clinical manifestations: Recurrent onsets of diarrhea with white milky masses or undigested food in stool, and often occurring after eating. Other manifestations include lassitude, emaciation, sallow complexion, sleeping with the eyes open, a pale tongue with white coating, and a weak pulse.

Analysis: Deficiency of the spleen following prolonged diarrhea impairs its function of transportation and transformation and thereby results in recurrent onsets of diarrhea. Lassitude is the result of damp disturbance with deficiency of the spleen. Emaciation, sleeping with the eyes open, and sallowish complexion are caused by deficiency of spleen Qi, which means insufficient source of Qi and blood. A pale tongue with white coating, and a weak pulse are signs resulting from deficiency of spleen Yang.

Treatment

Chinese herbal medicine:

a. Retention of food.

Treatment principle: To aid digestion and relieve stagnation.

Recipe: Baohe Wan (Pill for Protecting Harmony).

Prescription:

10 g of Jiaoshanzha (Fructus Crataegi, burnt)

10 g of Jiaoshenqu (Massa Fermentata Medicinalis, burnt)

10 g of Chaomaiya (Fructus Hordei Germinatus, fried)
10 g of Chaolaifuzi (Semen Raphani, fried)
5 g of Chenpi (Pericarpium Citri Reticulatae)
10 g of Fuling (Poria)

Explanation: This prescription aids digestion and pacifies the stomach. Shanzha, Shenqu and Maiya assist digestion and invigorate the spleen. Chaolaifuzi and Chenpi aid digestion and regulate Qi. Fuling invigorates the spleen and dispels damp.

b. Damp-heat.

Treatment principle: To relieve exterior symptoms, raise body fluid, clear heat in the intestines, and resolve damp.

Recipe: Gegen Huangqin Huanglian Tang (Decoction of Radix Puerariae, Radix Scutellariae and Rhizoma Coptidis).

Prescription:

10 g of Gegen (Radix Puerariae)
10 g of Chaohuangqin (Radix Scutellariae, fried)
2 g of Chaohuanglian (Rhizoma Coptidis, fried)
5 g of Zhigancao (Radix Glycyrrhizae, treated)
20 g of Machixian (Herba Portulacae)
20 g of Tiexiancai (Herba Acalyph Australis)

Explanation: This prescription clears heat in the intestines and resolves damp. Gegen relieves exterior symptoms and sends body fluid upward. Huangqin and Huanglian clear damp heat in the stomach and intestines. Gancao pacifies the middle Jiao with its sweet property. Machixian and Tiexiancai strengthen the effect of clearing heat in the intestines.

If damp predominates with a white and sticky tongue coating, herbs are prescribed on the basis of Huoxiang Zhengqi San (Powder of Herba Agastachis for Normalizing Qi).

c. Deficiency of the spleen.

Treatment principle: To invigorate the spleen and benefit Qi.

Recipe: Shen Ling Baizhu San (Powder of Radix Ginseng, Poria and Rhizoma Atractylodis Macrocephalae).

Prescription:

10 g of Taizishen (Radix Pseudostellariae)

10 g of Shanyao (Rhizoma Dioscoreae)

10 g of Chaobaizhu (Rhizoma Atractylodis Macrocephalae, fried)

10 g of Fuling (Poria)

10 g of Chaoyiren (Semen Coicis, fried)

10 g of Chaobiandou (Semen Dolichoris Album, fried)

2 g of Sharen (Fructus Amomi)

5 g of Paojiangtan (Rhizoma Zingiberis, charred)

Explanation: This prescription benefits Qi, invigorates the spleen, pacifies the stomach, and dispels damp through urine. Taizishen and Shanyao benefit Qi and invigorate the spleen. Baizhu, Fuling, Chaoyiren and Chaobiandou invigorate the spleen and dispel damp through urine. Sharen regulates Qi and invigorates the spleen. Paojiangtan warms spleen Yang.

Acupuncture treatment:

a. Excess syndromes (including retention of food and damp-heat).

Treatment principle: To pacify the stomach and relieve stagnation for retention of food; and to clear heat in the intestines and resolve damp for damp-heat. Points are selected from the Stomach and Ren channels and needled with the reducing method.

Prescription: Tianshu (St. 25) 1, Zhongwan (Ren 12)

1, Qihai (Ren 6) 1, Zusanli (St. 36) L.

Explanation: Tianshu (St. 25), the Front-Mu Point of the large intestine, and Zhongwan (Ren 12), the Front-Mu Point of the Stomach, combine to clear heat in the intestines and pacify the middle Jiao. Qihai (Ren 6) regulates Qi and relieves stagnation. Zusanli (St. 36) pacifies the stomach and checks diarrhea.

Points according to symptoms and signs:

Fever: Quchi (L.I. 11) L, Neiting (St. 44) L.

Restlessness and thirst: Shenmen (H. 7) 1, Zhaohai (K. 6) 1.

b. Deficiency syndromes (deficiency of the spleen).

Treatment principle: To invigorate the spleen, benefit Qi and check diarrhea. Needling with the reinforcing method is combined with moxibustion.

Prescription: Pishu (U.B. 20) T, Dachangshu (U.B. 25) T, Tianshu (St. 25) IX, Qihai (Ren 6) IX, Zusanli (St. 36) TX, Taibai (Sp. 3) TX.

Explanation: Tianshu (St. 25) and Dachangshu (U.B. 25), the Front-Mu and Back-Shu points of the large intestine, combine to regulate the function of the large intestine. Pishu (U.B. 20), Taibai (Sp. 3) and Zusanli (St. 36) invigorate the function of the spleen in transportation and transformation, and check diarrhea. Qihai (Ren 6) regulates Qi and relieves stagnation.

Other therapies:

a. Ear acupuncture.

Points: Small Intestine, Large Intestine, Stomach, Spleen, Sympathetic Nerve, Ear-Shenmen.

Method: These points are treated with either needling or implantation of rape seeds on both sides.

b. Moxibustion.

Points: Pishu (U.B. 20), Weishu (U.B. 21), Shenmen (H.

7), Guanyuan (Ren 4), Zusanli (St. 36).

Method: Move the moxa-stick up and down like sparrow feeding above each point for 3-5 minutes until the local area becomes red.

Discussion

Prolonged diarrhea damages Yin and Yang. In the case of damage of Yin, the method of nourishing Yin with sour and sweet herbs is adopted in herbal treatment; while in acupuncture treatment, the following points are needled with the even method: Pishu (U.B. 20) 1, Tianshu (St. 25) 1, Qihai (Ren 6) 1, Zusanli (St. 36) 1, Sanyinjiao (Sp. 6) 1, Zhaohai (K. 6) 1. In the case of damage of Yang, the method of recapturing Yang and rescuing the collapsing state is adopted in herbal treatment; while in acupuncture treatment, the following points are selected: Pishu (U.B. 20) IX, Zusanli (St. 36) 1, Mingmen (Du 4) X, Guanyuan (Ren 4) X, and Shenque (Ren 8), to which indirect moxibustion with salt is applied.

In the treatment of infantile diarrhea, food control is essential. In mild cases, feed the baby with less quantities of food or milk. In severe cases, the sick baby should not eat anything for 8-12 hours. When pathological conditions improve, food which can be easily digested is given such as a small amount of milk or rice soup. The supply of body fluid should be ensured during fasting.

For prophylaxis, the baby should be fed properly at definite hours of the day with a fixed quantity. Mother's milk is the preferable food. The quantity of other foods should increase gradually along with the adaptability of the spleen and stomach of the baby. For older children, they should pay attention to environmental and personal hygiene, wash their hands before meals or after visiting the toilet, and not to eat spoilt food.

7. Gan Syndrome (Malnutrition)

Infantile Gan syndrome is a chronic disease resulting from deficiency of the spleen and stomach, which deprives the Zang-Fu organs of nourishment. Characterized by emaciation, sallow complexion, sparse hair, abnormal appetite and bowel movements, this disease often occurs in children under three years of age. Due to slow onset and long duration of the disease, the growth and development of the sick child are retarded. Weakness of body resistance in a prolonged case will cause complications, and thereby make the pathological condition even worse.

The principal pathogenesis of this disease is dysfunction of the spleen and stomach, which results from improper feeding or lack of recuperation following a prolonged illness. The spleen and stomach are diseased in Gan syndrome no matter what the causative factor is. The early stage of the disease presents dysharmony of the spleen and stomach; the middle stage manifests as deficiency of the spleen with retention of food or intestinal parasites; and the late stage exhibits deficiency of the spleen complicated with deficiency of Qi and blood.

Gan syndrome in a prolonged case can possibly affect other Zang-Fu organs. Disorders of the spleen affecting the liver is commonly seen. The liver opens into the eye. When the liver is deprived of nourishment and liver blood becomes insufficient due to disorders of the spleen, the eyes will not be able to be well nourished. As a result, a condition called eye Gan syndrome manifesting as night blindness and slight corneal opacity will ensue. A prolonged spleen disorder also implies dysfunction in transportation and transformation with the result of overflow of water and damp. Subsequently, a condition called Gan edema will occur. If deficiency of the spleen does not allow its performance of the function in controlling blood, blood extravasation will happen and thereby ecchymoses and bleeding will follow.

Differentiation

a. Dysharmony of the spleen and stomach.

Clinical manifestations: Slight emaciation, yellowish complexion, anorexia or voracious appetite, alternate loose stool and dry constipation, lassitude, irritability, a sticky tongue coating, and a forceful pulse.

Explanation: This is the early stage of Gan syndrome and therefore is mild. Dysharmony of the spleen and stomach impairs the function of the stomach in receiving food, and the function of the spleen in transportation and transformation. Thereby anorexia, voracious appetite, alternate loose stool and dry constipation are possible. Dysfunction of the spleen in absorbing food essence to nourish the body gives rise to emaciation and yellowish complexion. Deficiency of the spleen and hyperactivity of the liver explain irritability. Deficiency of the spleen with excess of damp is the cause of a sticky tongue coating.

b. Deficiency of the spleen with retention of food or intestinal parasites.

Clinical manifestations: Pronounced emaciation, sallow complexion, sparse hair, pot-belly with exposed veins in severe cases, lassitude, restlessness, reduced appetite or overeating with excessive amount of stool, discharge of intestinal parasites through anus, abnormal movements such as kneading the eyebrow, picking the nose, biting the fingers, and grinding the teeth, possibly preference for eating uncooked rice or even earth, a pale tongue with yellow and sticky coating, and a weak pulse.

Explanation: This syndrome is more severe than and follows on dysharmony of the spleen and stomach. Deficiency of the spleen complicated with retention of food or intestinal parasites injures the source of Qi and blood and thereby deprives the skin and muscles of nourishment with the result of emaciation and sallow complexion. Deficiency of blood leads to yellow and sparse hair, which is a part of blood. Disturbance of the stomach and intestines by parasites causes retarded circulation of Qi and also gives rise to pot-belly, reduced appetite, or preference for eating unusual food. Overeating with excessive amounts of stool is due to hyperactivity of the stomach and weakness of the spleen. Deficiency of the spleen stirs liver fire and thereby results in restlessness and abnormal movements.

c. Deficiency of the spleen complicated with deficiency of Qi and blood.

Clinical manifestations: Extreme emaciation, sallow complexion, dry and withered skin peeling off easily like an old man, disappearance of the muscles in the buttocks and thigh with the bones wrapped by skin, lassitude, crying without tears or strength, concave abdomen, anorexia, loose stool or constipation, dry lips and mouth, a pale and delicate or red tongue with peeled coating, and a weak pulse. Ecchymoses may be present all over the body in severe cases, and prostration is possible.

Explanation: This syndrome is the most severe, and is present at the late stage of the disease. Deficiency of the spleen and stomach deprives the skin and muscles of nourishment, and thereby gives rise to extreme emaciation and appearance of a little old man. Deficiency of Qi and blood accompanied by exhaustion of body fluid results in dry and withered skin and hair. Qi failing to control blood is the cause of ecchymoses. Prostration is the consequence of deficiency of both Qi and blood.

Treatment

Chinese herbal medicine:

a. Dysharmony of the spleen and stomach.

Treatment principle: To harmonize the spleen and stomach and invigorate their function in transportation and transformation.

Recipe: Zisheng Jianpi Wan (Pill for Generating Vitality and Invigorating the Spleen).

Prescription:

10 g of Shanyao (Rhizoma Dioscoreae)

10 g of Jiaoshanzha (Fructus Crataegi, burnt)

10 g of Chaoyiren (Semen Coicis, fried)

10 g of Chaobaizhu (Rhizoma Atractylodis Macrocephalae, fried)

10 g of Fuling (Poria)

10 g of Huoxiang (Herba Agastachis)

10 g of Chaozhishi (Fructus Aurantii Immaturus, fried)

10 g of Chaomaiya (Fructus Hordei Germinatus, fried)

Explanation: This prescription invigorates the function of the spleen in transportation and transformation. Therefore, it is indicated in dysharmony of the spleen and stomach and retentioon of food. Shanyao and Shanzha invigorate the spleen. Yiren, Fuling and Baizhu also invigorate the spleen. Huoxiang and Maiya pacify the stomach and invigorate the spleen. Zhishi regulates Qi and relieves stagnation.

b. Deficiency of the spleen with retention of food or intestinal parasites.

Treatment principle: To relieve stagnation and regulate the spleen.

Recipe: Ganji San (Powder for Relieving Stagnation).

Prescription:

5 g of Zhijineijin (Endothelium Corneum Gigeriae Galli, treated)

10 g of Chaoshenque (Massa Fermentata Medicinalis, fried)

10 g of Chaomaiya (Fructus Hordei Germinatus, fried)

5 g of Cangzhu (Rhizoma Atractylodis)

2 g of Sharen (Fructus Amomi)

3 g of Huhuanglian (Rhizoma Picrorhizae)

Explanation: This prescription regulates the spleen and stomach, relieves stagnation and kills parasites. Zhijineijin, Shenque and Maiya relieve stagnation. Cangzhu and Sharen resolve damp, invigorate the spleen and promote digestion. Huhuanglian relieves restlessness and kills parasites.

c. Deficiency of the spleen complicated with deficiency of Qi and blood.

Treatment principle: To tonify the spleen and benefit Qi.

Recipe: Shen Ling Baizhu San (Powder of Radix Ginseng, Poria and Rhizoma Atractylodis Macrocephalae).

Prescription:

10 g of Chaodangshen (Radix Codonopsis Pilosulae, fried)

10 g of Shanyao (Rhizoma Dioscoreae)

10 g of Chaolianrou (Semen Nelumbinis, fried)

10 g of Chaobaizhu (Rhizoma Atractylodis Macrocephalae, fried)

10 g of Chaoyiren (Semen Coicis, fried)

10 g of Chaobiandou (Semen Dolichoris Album, fried)

10 g of Fuling (Poria)

2 g of Sharen (Fructus Amomi)

Explanation: This prescription invigorates the spleen, benefits Qi, pacifies the stomach and dispels damp through urine. It is indicated in Gan syndrome due to deficiency of Qi of the spleen and stomach or complication of damp as well. Dashen, Shanyao and Lianrou are three main herbs acting to benefit Qi, invigorate the spleen, pacify the stomach and check diarrhea. Baizhu, Fuling, Yiren and Biandou are secondary herbs acting to invigorate the spleen and dispel damp through urine. As adjuvants, Zhigancao benefits Qi and pacifies the middle Jiao; and Sharen pacifies the stomach, invigorates the spleen, regulates Qi and relaxes the chest.

d. Treatment of complicated syndromes.

1) Gan syndrome involving the eye.

The clinical manifestations include dryness of the eyes, photophobia, and in severe cases, corneal opacity. This syndrome is due to disorders of the spleen affecting the liver, and giving rise to deficiency of liver Yin and flaring up of liver fire. The method of smoothing and nourishing the liver is used in the treatment by applying Shihu Yeguang Wan (Pill of Herba Dendrobii for Night Brightness).

2) Gan edema.

The clinical manifestations include systemic edema, scanty urine, pale complexion, a pale and delicate tongue with thin and white coating. This syndrome is due to deficiency of the spleen, which produces overflow of water and damp. The method of invigorating the spleen, warming Yang and discharging water is adopted with the emphasis laid on the spleen in the treatment. The applicable recipe is Wuling San (Poria Powder in Five Ingredients). Snakeheaded fish and carp are recommendable as dietary therapy.

Acupuncture treatment:

Needle Zhongwan (Ren 12) 1, Tianshu (St. 25) 1, Qihai (Ren 6) 1 and Zusanli (St. 36) 1 with moderate stimulation . The needles are not retained. Treatment is given once a day for 5-6 days. If this method is not effective, apply moxibustion to these four points plus Pishu (U.B. 20) and Shenshu (U.B. 23) as well.

Points according to symptoms and signs:

a. Dysharmony of the spleen and stomach: Pishu (U.B. 20) T, Ganshu (U.B. 18) T, Zhongwan (Ren 12) 1, Tianshu (St. 25) 1, Zusanli (St. 36) 1, Taichong (Liv. 3) 1.

b. Deficiency of the spleen with retention of food and parasites: Pishu (U.B. 20) T, Weishu (U.B. 21) T, Zhongwan (Ren 12) 1, Qihai (Ren 6) 1, Baichongwo (Extra.) 1, Zusanli (St. 36) 1.

c. Deficiency of the spleen complicated with deficiency of Qi and blood: Baihui (Du 20) X, Ganshu (U.B. 18) T, Pishu (U.B. 20) T, Tianshu (St. 25) 1, Guanyuan (Ren 4) TX, Zusanli (St. 36) T.

Other therapies:

A. Needling Sifeng (Extra.).

Prick Sifeng (Extra.) on both hands 0.5-1.0 inch with a three-edged needle. Squeeze out a small amount of yellow fluid from the acupuncture holes after withdrawing the needle, and then dry it out with sterilized cotton balls. Treatment is given once every other day. This method invigorates the spleen and relieves stagnation.

This method is applied from the sacrum up to Dazhui (Du 14) six times. When doing the third and fourth manoeuvres, lift with the wrist force the muscular ridge five to six times in the area above the waist. After the end of the sixth manoeuvre, push and press Mingmen (Du 4) towards Shenshu (U.B. 23) on both sides with the thumbs. This method regulates the spleen and stomach, clears channels and relieves stagnation.

b. Incision.

This method is usually applied to the middle area of the thenar eminence of the left hand. Only one operation is performed on the same baby, while the chance of two operations is slim. For details, refer to Chapter III.

Discussion

It is important to regulate the diet according to the pathological conditions in order to improve nourishment supply of the sick baby. Food of good quality which can be easily digested is recommended.

For prophylaxis, mother's milk is preferred. If mother's milk is not sufficient, feed the baby with cow milk or milk powder. The quantity of other foods with different types of nutritive value should increase gradually along with the increase of the baby's age in order to meet the needs for rapid growth and development of the body.

8. Convulsion

Convulsion may be caused by many factors in various diseases. Characterized by violent irregular movements of the limbs and body, and mental cloudiness, this disease occurs in all four seasons, more commonly in children under five years of age. The younger the children are, the higher the incidence of the disease will be. The incidence decreases gradually in children above seven years of age. Since the disease occurs suddenly with pathological conditions becoming critical rapidly, it threatens the life of children. That is why convulsion was listed as one of the four major pediatric diseases by medical scholars of all ages.

There are two categories of convulsion, acute convulsion manifesting as a syndrome of the excess type, and chronic convulsion manifesting as a syndrome of the deficiency type.

Acute convulsion

Acute convulsion is caused by invasion of external pathogenic factors including pestilential factors, and by retention of food or turbid phlegm in the interior, which blocks the clear cavity. The principal causative factors include heat, phlegm and wind, which influence each other. The heart and liver are mainly diseased.

Differentiation

Acute convulsion is usually the consequence of a febrile disease due to invasion by external pathogenic factors. It is necessary to differentiate whether the pathogenic factors are on the exterior of the body or in the interior. The former is mild while the latter is severe.

a. Invasion of external pathogenic factors.

Clinical manifestations: Fever, coughing, runny nose, severe headache, inflamed throat, convulsion of the four. limbs when fever is high, staring upward, lockjaw, a red tongue tip with thin and white or slightly yellow coating, and a superficial and rapid pulse. Convulsion stops as soon as fever subsides.

Analysis: This syndrome is due to invasion of the lung

by external pathogenic wind-heat. This explains fever, coughing and runny nose. Upward disturbance of heat in the lung and stomach gives rise to inflamed throat. Since both spirit and Qi of children are weak, and their tendons and channels are not strong, persistent high fever will lead to convulsion. Fever subsides after sweating, because the pathogenic factors are lodged on the exterior of the body. Convulsion stops at the same time. A red tongue tip with white or yellow coating, and a superficial and rapid pulse are both signs of invasion of the body surface by heat.

b. Retention of food and phlegm in the interior.

Clinical manifestations: The early stage of the syndrome presents anorexia, vomiting, abdominal pain, constipation, fever or absence of fever, dull expression, abdominal distension and fullness. Coma and convulsion soon follow accompanied by gurgling with sputum. The tongue coating is dirty and sticky, and the pulse is wiry and rolling.

Analysis: This syndrome often occurs in older children after voracious eating or intake of unclean food, either of which causes retention of food and thereby impairs the function of the spleen in transportation and transformation with the result of production of phlegm. Dysfunction of the stomach in descending is the cause of vomiting. Retardation of Qi circulation produces obstruction, which explains abdominal distension and pain, and constipation. Retention of food and phlegm produces heat, which manifests as fever. Upward movement of phlegm-heat stirs liver wind and thereby causes mental cloudiness and convulsion. A dirty and sticky tongue coating, and a wiry and rolling pulse are both signs of turbid phlegm.

103

Treatment

Phlegm should be dispelled in the treatment of convulsion. Wind should be eliminated in order to dispel phlegm. Fever should be relieved in order to eliminate wind. And pathogenic factors should be eliminated in order to relieve fever.

Chinese herbal medicine:

a. Invasion of external pathogenic factors.

Treatment principle: To eliminate wind, clear heat and dispel phlegm.

Recipe: Yinqiao San (Powder of Flos Lonicerae and Fructus Forsythiae)

Prescription:

10 g of Yinhua (Flos Lonicerae)

10 g of Lianqiao (Fructus Forsythiae)

5 g of Bohe (Herba Menthae)

10 g of Niubangzi (Fructus Arctii)

5 g of Chanyi (Periostracum Cicadae)

10 g of Zhijiangcan (Bombyx Batryticatus, treated)

10 g of Gouteng (Ramulus Uncariae cum Uncis)

5 g of Changpu (Rhizoma Acori Graminei)

Explanation: This prescription disperses wind-heat and relieves toxins. Yinhua and Lianqiao clear heat and relieve toxins. Bohe and Niubangzi disperse wind and ease the throat. Chanyi and Jiangcan eliminate wind and relieve convulsion. Gouteng, an important herb in the treatment of disorders of the Heart and Liver channels, clears heat and calms wind. Changpu dispels phlegm and promotes mental resuscitation.

As for acute convulsion due to invasion by pestilential factors, refer to the treatment of acute infectious febrile diseases and toxic bacillary dysentery.

b. Retention of food and phlegm.

Treatment principle: To aid digestion, resolve phlegm and regain mental clarity.

Recipe: Yushu Dan (Jade Pivot Pill)

Prescription: Yushu Dan, to be taken twice a day, 0.6-1.0 g each time for babies.

Explanation: Since this medicine dispels the turbidity, relieves toxins, regains mental clarity and checks vomiting, it is a very important medicine for first aid in the treatment of diseases of internal medicine. Its principal indication covers diseases caused by damp, heat, summer heat and turbid phlegm, especially those marked by mental disturbance, convulsion, and a moist, thick and sticky or dirty and sticky tongue coating.

Acupuncture treatment:

a. Invasion of external pathogenic factors.

Treatment principle: To relieve exterior symptoms, clear heat, calm wind and resolve phlegm. Acupuncture with the reducing method is applied.

Prescription: Dazhui (Du 14) 1, Quchi (L.I. 11) L, Hegu (L.I. 4) L, Fenglong (St. 40) L.

Points according to symptoms and signs:

High fever: Shixuan (Extra.), to be pricked to cause bleeding.

Convulsion: Taichong (Liv. 3) through to Yongquan (K. 1) L.

Lockjaw: Xiaguan (St. 7) 1, Jiache (St. 6) 1.

Headache: Taiyang (Extra.) 1.

Explanation: Dazhui (Du 14), Quchi (L.I. 11), Hegu (L.I. 4) and Shixuan (Extra.) relieve exterior symptoms and clear heat. Needling Taichong (Liv. 3) through to Yongquan (K. 1) suppresses liver wind. Fenglong (St. 40) resolves phlegm.

b. Retention of food and phlegm.

Treatment principle: To refresh the brain, regain mental clarity, pacify the stomach and resolve phlegm. Acupuncture with the reducing method is applied.

Prescription: Baihui (Du 20) L, Renzhong (Du 26) L, Neiguan (P. 6) L, Tianshu (St. 25) l, Fenglong(St. 40) L.

Points according to symptoms and signs:

Fever: Quchi (L.I. 11) L.

Abdominal pain and constipation: Qihai (Ren 6) l, Tianshu (St. 25) l.

Dull expression: Yintang (Extra.) l.

Gurgling with sputum: Tiantu (Ren 22) l.

Explanation: Baihui (Du 20) and Renzhong (Du 26) refresh the brain and regain mental clarity. Neiguan (P. 6) checks vomiting and pacifies the stomach. Tianshu (St. 25) regulates the intestines and relieves stagnation. Fenglong (St. 40) resolves phlegm.

Other therapies:

a. Ear acupuncture.

Points: Sympathetic Nerve, Ear-Shenmen, Subcortex, Brain Point, Heart.

Method: These points are needled with strong stimulation. The needles are manipulated once every 10 minutes during an hour's retention.

Chronic convulsion

Chronic convulsion results from injury of Yin of the liver and kidney due to acute convulsion, or from prolonged vomiting and diarrhea, which weakens the spleen and stomach and subsequently leads to deficiency of Yang of the spleen and kidney. Either deficiency of Yin of the liver and kidney or deficiency of Yang of the spleen and kidney produces wind. Therefore, chronic convulsion mainly involves the spleen, liver and kidney.

Differentiation

Chronic convulsion is due to wind of the deficiency type. There are following two syndromes.

a. Deficiency of Yin of the liver and kidney.

Clinical manifestations: Emaciation, withered spirit, restlessness, low-grade fever, a heat sensation in the palms and soles, sweating, tremor of the four limbs or rigidity of the body and limbs, dry stool, a deep-red tongue with scanty moisture and peeled coating, and a thready and rapid pulse.

Analysis: This syndrome follows on acute convulsion, which persists over a long period of time, and gives rise to deficiency of Yin of the liver and kidney. Deficiency of Yin produces internal heat, which explains low-grade fever, restlessness, a heat sensation in the palms and soles, excessive sweating, emaciation and withered spirit. Deficiency of Qi and blood deprives the tendons and channels of nourishment, and thereby wind of the deficiency type is stirred in the interior. This is the cause of tremor of the four limbs or rigidity of the body and limbs. Dry stool, a red tongue with scanty moisture and peeled coating, and a thready and rapid pulse are all signs of exhaustion of Yin fluid.

b. Deficiency of Yang of the spleen and kidney.

Clinical manifestations: Pale complexion, indifference, sweating, cold limbs, whites of the eyes revealed when asleep, twitching of hands and feet, clear urine, loose stool, a pale tongue with thin and white coating, and a deep and thready or feeble and weak pulse.

Analysis: This syndrome is due to deficiency of Yang of the spleen and kidney and deficiency of Yuan Qi (congenital Qi). The normal functioning of the spleen in transportation and transformation needs warmth and nourishment of kidney Yang, while kidney Yang relies on spleen Yang for continuous production. Deficiency of Yang to the spleen and kidney produces internal cold and thereby gives rise to a condition of excess of Yin with deficiency of Yang. At the late stage of chronic convulsion, the critical signs of collapse of Yang Qi are present.

Treatment

The principle "The reinforcing method is applied for syndromes of the deficiency type" is observed. In these two syndromes, there is no convulsion to relieve, nor there is wind to eliminate. Therefore, oral administration of herbs which suppress convulsion and eliminate wind would do a lot of harm to the patient.

Chinese herbal medicine:

a. Deficiency of Yin of the liver and kidney.

Treatment principle: To tonify water, nourish wood, calm wind, and subdue Yang.

Recipe: Dadingfeng Zhu (Precious Decoction for Ceasing Wind).

Prescription:

10 g of Ejiao (Colla Corii Asini), to be melted and taken with water separately

10 g of Shengdi (Radix Rehmanniae)

10 g of Maidong (Radix Ophiopogonis)

10 g of Baishao (Radix Paeoniae Alba)

10 g of Guiban (Plastrum Testudinis)

10 g of Biejia (Carapax Trionycis)

10 g of Muli (Concha Ostreae)

5 g of Wuweizi (Fructus Schisandrae)

5 g of Gancao (Radix Glycyrrhizae)

Explanation: This prescription is most suitable to deficiency of Yin of the liver and kidney complicated with stirring of wind in the interior. Ejiao nourishes Yin and calms wind. Shengdi, Maidong and Baishao nourish Yin and ease the liver. Guiban, Biejia and Muli produce Yin and subdue Liver Yang. Zhigancao and Wuweizi produce Yin with their sweat and sour nature.

b. Deficiency of Yang of the spleen and kidney.

Treatment principle: To benefit fire, produce earth, recapture Yang and rescue the collapsing state.

Recipe: Guzhen Tang (Decoction for Consolidating Yang).

Prescription:

10 g of Renshen (Radix Ginseng)

10 g of Shufuzi (Radix Aconiti Praeparata)

1 g of Rougui (Cortex Cinnamomi)

10 g of Longgu (Os Draconis)

10 g of Muli (Concha Ostreae)

5 g of Zhigancao (Radix Glycyrrhizae, treated)

10 g of Zhihuangqi (Radix Astragali, treated)

10 g of Chaobaizhu (Rhizoma Atractylodis Macrocephalae, fried)

Explanation: This prescription warms and tonifies the spleen and kidney, recaptures Yang and rescues the collapsing state. Renshen tonifies Yuanqi (congenital Qi). Fuzi and Rougui tonify fire and aid Yang. Longgu and Muli subdue liver Yang and avoid the collapsing state. Zhihuangqi, Chaobaizhu and Zhigancao benefit Qi and invigorate the spleen.

Acupuncture treatment:

a. Deficiency of Yin of the liver and kidney.

Treatment principle: To nourish Yin and subdue Yang. Acupuncture with the reinforcing method is applied.

Prescription: Ganshu (U.B. 18) T, Shenshu (U.B. 23) T,

Yinxi (H. 6) 1, Shousanli (L.I. 10) 1, Yanglingquan (G.B. 34) 1, Fuliu (K. 7) 1, Taichong (Liv. 3) 1.

Explanation: Ganshu (U.B. 18), Shenshu (U.B. 23), Yinxi (H. 6) and Fuliu (K. 7) nourish the liver and kidney, and check sweating. Shousanli (L.I. 10), Yanglingquan (G.B. 34) and Taichong (Liv. 3) calm wind and suppress tremor.

b. Deficiency of Yang of the spleen and kidney.

Treatment principle: To invigorate the spleen, recapture Yang and rescue the collapsing state. Acupuncture with the reinforcing method is combined with moxibustion.

Prescription: Baihui (Du 20) 1, Yintang (Extra.) 1, Tianshu (St. 25) IX, Guanyuan (Ren 4) IX, Shenque (Ren 8) △ with salt, Zusanli (St. 36) T.

Explanation: Baihui (Du 20) and Yintang (Extra.) refresh the brain. Tianshu (St. 25) treated with both acupuncture and moxibustion warms the intestines and checks diarrhea. Guanyuan (Ren 4), Shenque (Ren 8) and Zusanli (St. 36) recapture Yang and rescue the collapsing state.

Discussion

Heat, phlegm, wind and violent jerking movements of the body are not only clinical characteristics, but also the etiological factors of acute convulsion. Although it originates from prolonged acute convulsion, chronic convulsion manifests differently. The acute one is of the excess type and marked by abrupt onset and violent manifestations. Convulsion should be relieved first by applying needling, massage and Chinese patent medicines. Other symptoms and signs will then be treated on the basis of differentiation of syndromes. The chronic convulsion is of the deficiency type. The emphasis in the treatment is laid on strengthening body resistance by prescribing herbs in the form of decoction, which is assisted by moxibustion and acupuncture with the reinforcing method.

At the time of convulsion, lay the child flat on the bed with the head resting on the side. Then unbutton the shirt to keep the respiratory tract free of obstruction. Then put tongue depressor wrapped with several layers of gauze in between the upper and lower teeth in order to avoid biting the tongue. Then administer oxygen to the child and suck sputum to prevent suffocation. To prevent bedsore, the sleeping position should change frequently for the sick child who has long rested on bed; and rub the body with a soft towel dipped in warm water so as to keep Qi and blood circulating smoothly.

9. Epilepsy

The local name of epilepsy is goat epileptic wind. As a paroxysmal mental disorder, epilepsy characteristically manifests as sudden collapse, loss of consciousness, staring upward, convulsion of the four limbs, spitting of white frothy saliva or making a noise like a goat. Between epileptic attacks, there are intervals, at which the patient looks healthy. This disease often occurs in older children. The sick child with frequent attacks usually has retarded intelligence.

The causative factors before birth include fetal shock and heredity, while blockage of the heart and mind by persistent phlegm is the cause after birth. Since phlegm accumulates and disperses, and wind moves and ceases alternately, there are intermittent epileptic seizures.

111

Differentiation

It is necessary to differentiate epilepsy due to wind and epilepsy due to phlegm. If convulsion is the main symptom at the time of the attack, epilepsy is due to wind. If the patient falls with much sputum in the throat during the attack, epilepsy is due to phlegm.

a. Epilepsy due to wind.

Clinical manifestations: Abrupt onset of severe convulsion, rigidity of the limbs and body, blue complexion, coma, lockjaw, staring upward or sideway, twitching of the mouth, spitting of saliva, a red tongue tip and border with a yellow or white coating, and a wiry pulse.

Analysis: This syndrome is due to retention of phlegm, which transforms into fire and produces wind. Wind and phlegm disturb upward, clouding the heart and mind. This explains coma and convulsion. Wind and phlegm invading the channels and collaterals is the cause of rigidity of the limbs and body, lockjaw and staring upward. Upward accumulation of wind and phlegm gives rise to twitching of the mouth and spitting of saliva. Blue complexion, a red tongue tip, and a wiry pulse are all signs due to internal disturbance of wind and phlegm.

b. Epilepsy due to phlegm.

Clinical manifestations: Sudden collapse, mental cloudiness, staring forward like an idiot, less pronounced convulsion of the four limbs or the body, gurgling with sputum in the throat, spitting of sputum-like fluid at the corner of the mouth, a thick and sticky tongue coating, and a rolling pulse.

Analysis: This syndrome is due to retention of wind and phlegm in the interior of the body, and often occurs in older children. Upward disturbance of turbid phlegm clouds the heart, and thereby gives rise to sudden collapse, mental cloudiness, spitting of sputum-like fluid, and gurgling with sputum in the throat. Retention of the pathogenic factor in the Liver Channel causes stagnation of liver Qi, which, accompanied by wind-phlegm, results in staring forward and convulsion, though convulsion is not severe. A thick and sticky tongue coating and a rolling pulse are both signs of retention of excessive turbid phlegm in the interior.

Treatment

To dispel phlegm and calm wind is the general principle of treatment. Since this disease presents intermittent seizures, treatment should continue for a long period of time.

***Chinese herbal medicine*:**

a. Epilepsy due to wind.

Treatment principle: To calm wind and relieve convulsion.

Recipe: Jiawei Zhijing San (Powder for Relieving Convulsion with Additional Ingredients).

Prescription:

20 g of Zhiquanxie (Scorpio, treated)

20 g of Wugong (Scolopendra)

20 g of Zhijiangcan (Bombyx Batryticatus, treated)

20 g of Chendanxing (Arisaema cum Bile, preserved)

10 g of Zhiyuanzhi (Radix Polygalae, treated)

20 g of Fanshuiyujin (Radix Curcumae, alum water treated)

Explanation: Chendanxing and Zhiyuanzhi resolve phlegm and regain mantal clarity. Zhiquanxie, Wugong and Zhijiancan eliminate wind, remove obstruction in the channels and relieve convulsion. Fangshuiyujin resolves phlegm and relieves stagnation. This recipe should be administered for a long time.

b. Epilepsy due to phlegm.

Treatment principle: To dispel phlegm and relieve epilepsy.

Recipe: Zhuli Datan Wan (Bamboo Juice Pill for Dispelling Phlegm).

Prescription:

20 ml of Zhuli (Bamboo Juice obtained with heating)

10 g of Mengshi (Chlorite-schist)

2 g of Chenxiang (Lignum Aquilariae Resinatum)

5 g of Changpu (Rhizoma Acori Graminei)

5 g of Danxing (Arisaema cum Bile)

10 g of Fanshuiyujin (Radix Curcumae, alum water treated)

1 g of Quanxie (Scorpio), to be ground into powder and taken separately once a day

1 g of Jiangcan (Bombyx Batryticatus), to be ground into powder and taken separately once a day

Explanation: This prescription resolves and dispels phlegm, calms wind and regains mental clarity. Zhuli and Mengshi dispel persistent phlegm. Chengxiang sends perverse Qi downward rapidly. Changpu, Danxing and Fanshuiyujin dispel phlegm and regain mental clarity. Quanxie and Jiangcan relieve epilepsy and calm wind.

Acupuncture treatment:

a. Epilepsy due to wind.

Treatment principle: To calm wind, resolve phlegm and relieve convulsion. Acupuncture with the reducing method is applied.

Prescription: Baihui (Du 20) L, Renzhong (Du 26) L, Shenmen (H. 7) 1, Fenglong (St. 40) L, Taichong (Liv. 3) L.

Points according to symptoms and signs:

Lockjaw: Xiaguan (St. 7) 1, Jiache (St. 6) 1.

Staring upward: Zanzhu (U.B. 2) 1.

Explanation: Baihui (Du 20), Renzhong (Du 26), Shenmen (H. 7) and Taichong (Liv. 3) calm the mind and relieve convulsion. Fenglong (St. 40) resolves phlegm.

b. *Epilepsy due to phlegm.*

Treatment principle: To resolve phlegm and relieve epilepsy. Acupuncture with the reducing method is applied.

Prescription: Baihui (Du 20) L , Renzhong (Du 26) L, Shenmen (H. 7) 1, Yanglingquan (G.B. 34) L, Fenglong (St. 40) L, Taichong (Liv. 3) L.

Points according to symptoms and signs:

Gurgling with sputum: Tiantu (Ren 22) 1.

Salivation: Dicang (St. 4) 1, Chengjiang (Ren 24) 1.

Explanation: Baihui (Du 20), Renzhong (Du 26) and Shenmen (H. 7) calm the mind and refresh the brain. Fenglong (St. 40) resolves phlegm. Yanglingquan (G.B. 34) and Taichong (Liv. 3) relieve convulsion.

Other therapies:

Ear acupuncture.

Points: Stomach, Subcortex, Ear-Shenmen, Heart, Occiput, Brain Point.

Method: Choose two to three points at one sitting. Strong stimulation is given and needles are retained for 30 minutes.

Discussion

Epilepsy at the initial stage is mostly of the excess type, while that of long duration presents a complicated syndrome of Ben (underlying cause) deficiency and Biao (symptoms and signs) excess. At the time of seizure, Biao is treated by dispelling phlegm and calming wind. As key herbs for dispelling wind, Quanxie (Scorpio), Wugong (Scolopendra) and Jiangcan (Bombyx Batryticatus) have proved effective in the treatment of epilepsy of all types. In the treatment of prolonged epilepsy, recipes for nourishing the heart and calming the mind are used as well such as Gan Mai Dazao Tang (Decoction of Treated Radix Glycyrrhizae, Wheat and Fructus Ziziphi Jujubae), to which Longgu (Os Draconis), Muli (Concha Ostreae), Changpu (Rhizoma Acori Graminei), Yuanzhi (Radix Polygalae) and Baiziren (Semen Biotae) are added in order to treat both Biao and Ben.

See to it that the child does not eat a lot, because voracious eating may induce new seizures. The sick child should avoid mental irritation such as worry, fear and fright.

10. Intestinal Parasites

Common intestinal parasites of children include roundworm, pinworm, hookworm and fasciolopsis. The incidence of roundworm is the highest.

Roundworm was known as "long worm" in ancient times. The symptoms and signs are not pronounced if the child has only a small number of roundworms. The child with a large number of roundworms presents such symptoms as emaciation, yellow complexion, abnormal appetite, abdominal pain around the umbilicus, and discharge of roundworms through vomiting or defecation. Intake of unclean food or eating with dirty hands may allow their eggs to enter the body via the mouth. The adult worms live in the small intestines.

Pinworm is locally called "thread worm" as it looks like a white thread end. The principal sign is itching around the anus at night. Taking in its eggs via the mouth is the route of infection. Superinfection may take place if the child with pinworms scratches the itching area around the anus with the hands and then eats with the dirty hands.

Hookworm is conventionally known as "lazy and yellow disease," and characteristically manifests as sallow or pale complexion, fatigue and edema, all of which are possibly accompanied by reduced appetite or pica, e.g., preference for eating uncooked rice and earth. This disease is induced by the skin of the child contacting the baby hookworms in the epidemic areas, e.g., walking with bare feet or sitting on the ground with exposed buttocks.

Fasciolopsiasis looks like a ginger slice, and is also called "red worm." The main clinical manifestations include abdominal pain, diarrhea, emaciation and sallow complexion. This disease is induced by eating water plants such as water caltrop and water chestnut with metacercaria.

Differentiation

Invasion of the body by parasites impairs digestive function of the spleen and stomach, and thereby produces damp-heat, which is a good condition for parasites to live in. At the same time, such symptoms as anorexia, pica, abdominal pain and unformed stool occur.

Prolonged intestinal parasites weaken the spleen and stomach so that food essence is not able to be absorbed; they also disturb vital energy of the stomach and intestines and consume Qi and blood. Subsequently, there will occur symptoms of deficiency of Qi and blood such as sallow complexion, edema, palpitation and shortness of breath.

Roundworm lives in the intestines thus blocking the middle Jiao and disturbing vital energy with the result of intermittent occurrence of abdominal pain. The upward and downward movements of a roundworm give rise to violent pain if it enters the biliary tract and to discharge of the worm through vomiting and cold limbs.

Treatment

Different methods are adopted to treat intestinal parasites. At the initial stage of ascariasis when the child is still strong, the method of treatment is to dispel roundworms directly. In a prolonged case, the spleen and stomach are regulated first so as to produce sufficient Qi and blood, and then the method of dispelling roundworms is used. Anyway, dispelling method is the main approach towards the treatment of intestinal parasites.

Chinese herbal medicine:

a. Ascariasis.

(1) Dispelling roundworm.

a) Shijunzi San (Fructus Quisqualis Powder), to be taken once daily on an empty stomach for 2-3 days in succession.

b) Chew and swallow fried meat of Fructus Quisqualis. See to it that the fried meat smells good and is not burnt. The daily dosage is one to two pieces (each piece weighs about 0.5 g) for each year of age with the total daily amount not exceeding 20 pieces. These pieces are taken in the early morning on an empty stomach. Two hours later, administer purgatives to the child. The procedure is repeated for two days. Then the child rests for seven days before another three days of oral administration of the above drugs. To avoid hiccup, don't drink hot fluid within an hour after taking these drugs. Oral administration of large amounts of these drugs may cause such symptoms as dizziness, vertigo, vomiting and hiccup. However, hiccup can be checked by taking 3-5 g of powder of sword bean which has been fried yellow.

(2) Calming roundworm.

Wumei Wan (Fructus Mume Pill), to be taken twice daily, 10 g each time for children from seven to twelve, 4-8 g for children between three and six. This recipe can be administered continuously for several days without any side-effects.

b. Oxyuriasis.

1) Anthelmintic powder. The dosage is calculated according to the formula (age $+1) \times 0.3$ g, with the total daily amount not exceeding 12 g. This medicine is taken three times a day, one hour before meals for seven days in succession.

2) Baibu Fen (Powder of Radix Stemonae), to be taken once daily on an empty stomach in the morning, 1 g for each year of age each time with the daily dosage not exceeding 8 g. This amount of powder can also be taken in two to three installments within two hours. The purgatives are administered two hours later. This continues for two days. The second course of oral administration for three days begins after a seven-day interval.

c. Ancylostomiasis.

1) Guanzhong Tang (Decoction of Rhizoma Cyrtomium).

This recipe consists of 30 g of Guanzhong (Rhizoma Cyrtomium), 15 g of Kuliangenpi (Cortex Meliae), 15 g of Zisu (Folium Perillae), and 15 g of Tujingjie (Herba Chenopodium). All these herbs are cooked for two hours until the broth becomes thick. Then obtain the broth through a filter. Add 2/3 of the amount of water for the first decoction to the cooked material. The new broth is formed after another two hours of cooking. Mix these two types of broth and concentrate it down to 30-60 ml, which is the daily dosage for an adult. The dosage for a child decreases accordingly. The preparation is taken in the morning.

2) Leiwan Fen (Omphalia Powder), to be mixed in boiling water and taken three times a day, 5 g daily for children from three to five, 10 g daily for children from six to nine, and 15 g daily for children from 11 to 14, either before or after meals for two to three days in succession.

d. Fasciolopsiasis.

Break 30 g of Binglang (Semen Arecae) into pieces, which are soaked in 500 ml of clean water for one night. Then cook them for two hours until the broth becomes thick. The entire broth is taken at one time on an empty stomach in the morning. The treatment continues for three days.

If a deficiency syndrome is presented, the stomach and spleen are regulated, and Qi and blood are tonified. To regulate the spleen and stomach, Xiang Sha Liujunzi Wan (Pill of Six Noble Ingredients plus Radix Aucklandiae and Fructus Amomi) or Jianpi Wan (Pill for Invigorating the Spleen) is administered. To tonify Qi and blood, Famu Wan (Lumberjack's Pill) or Bazhen Tang (Decoction of Eight Pearls) is recommended. All these patent medicines are taken after meals for one to two months.

Acupuncture treatment:

Intestinal parasites of children are mainly treated with herbal medicine. However, acupuncture assists the treatment by regulating the spleen and stomach, regulating Qi and relieving pain.

a. If the parasites are in the stomach, needle Neiguan (P. 6) 1, Zhongwan (Ren 12) 1 and Gongsun (Sp. 4) 1.

b. If the parasites are in the intestines, needle Tianshu (St. 25) 1, Qihai (Ren 6) 1 and Shangjuxu (St. 37) 1.

c. If the parasites are in the biliary tract, needle Riyue (G.B. 24) 1, Burong (St. 19) 1, Zhongwan (Ren 12) 1 and Dannangxie (Extra.) L.

Other therapies:

a. Treatment of intestinal obstruction due to ascariasis with Chinese massage therapy.

Administer 50-100 ml of vegetable oil to the sick child, and massage on the abdomen begins 1-1.5 hours later for the purpose of lubricating the roundworms and loosening the mass.

The operator stands on the right side of the child and massages the skin of the abdomen with talcum powder medium with the palm from light to heavy in a clockwise direction, namely, from the right lower quadrant to the right upper quadrant to the left upper quadrant and to the left lower quadrant. If the loosening of the parasitic mass is too slow, digging technique can help. Generally speaking, the parasitic mass disperses after 30-40 minutes of massage. At this time, the sick child will probably fall asleep due to alleviation of abdominal pain.

Intestinal obstruction due to ascariasis can be relieved after 30-40 minutes of massage. A large number of roundworms are discharged in 12-24 hours. Most of the patients can expect cure in 48 hours. Further examination is required and corresponding measures should be taken if fever or dehydration occurs.

b. Treatment of ascariasis in the biliary tract by pressing with the thumb on the inferior angle of the right scapula.

This method renders good therapeutic results. The sick child takes front sitting position with the shoulders drooping naturally. The operator presses heavily on the inferior angle of the right scapula of the patient with the flat of the right thumb. Pressing continues for one to three minutes after a sensation of soreness or distension appears. Then massage the area for a while. Treatment is given once daily.

To avoid a relapse, anthelmintics should be administered one week after the symptoms and signs have disappeared.

c. Treatment of ascariasis in the biliary tract with pushing and pressing techniques.

The patient takes supine position with the knees flexed. The operator stands on the right side of the patient. Put a small amount of talcum powder or vaseline on the flat of the right thumb, and then press with it on the tender area 3-4 cm below the xiphoid process on the upper abdomen (corresponding to the common bile duct) from light to heavy. The force of pressing should be endurable. The massage proceeds from pressing, pushing to releasing, and then the procedure is repeated seven to eight times. Then a sudden and heavy pressing and pushing method is adopted when the abdominal muscles are relaxed 20-40 manoeuvers are required at one treatment. Most patients may shout during the treatment, because the massage may create transient but violent pain. The operator then should keep pressing the painful spot until pain is relieved. At the same time other techniques of massage should discontinue. The alleviation of pain suggests the withdrawal of the roundworms from the biliary tract to the duodenum. Treatment discontinues then. If the roundworms have penetrated to the deep layer of the biliary tract, pain will not follow in one to two such treatments. This method, however, is still applicable in such conditions.

Massage should be applied gently and slowly if there occurs the palpable gall bladder and tenderness due to high internal pressure of the biliary tract or complicated infection. Pressing and pushing techniques are then performed on the gall bladder area towards the xyphoid process five to six times. Then press and push the area of the common bile duct 20-30 times. The procedure is repeated two to three times.

It is neccesary to establish correct diagnosis before pushing and pressing techniques are performed. This method of treatment is used while the stomach of the patient is empty, since the increased tension of a full stomach may create accident. This method is prohibited in the cases of gastric ulcer, gastric bleeding, and enlargement of the liver. Only experienced doctors are allowed to use this method.

Discussion

In the experience of medical scholars of all ages, the occurrence of blue spots in the sclera, white spots in the lips, red spots on the tongue and a geographic tongue may suggest intestinal parasites. But this is not absolute. Some of the above phenomena are possibly physiological.

It has proved more effective to use two or more anthelmintics at the same time than to use a single one. Generally, those anthelmintics which are effective, convenient to use, cheap, available and create less side-effects are chosen.

11. Edema

Edema is a common disease of children, and is accompanied by scanty urine. This disease may occur in all seasons, but that due to common cold or tonsillitis is more often seen in winter and spring, and that due to pathogenic toxins is more commonly present in summer and autumn. Generally, edema Yang in nature is of short duration, and the prognosis is good, while edema Yin in nature is of long duration with recurrent attacks, and thus the prognosis is poor.

Edema of children is principally caused by exposure to external pathogenic wind, retention of water and damp in the interior, and invasion of the interior of the body by pathogenic toxins, either of which impairs the function of the lung, spleen and kidney in regulating body fluid.

Nephritis and nephrosis are included in this discussion.

Differentiation

Differentiation is based on the acuteness of onset, duration of the disease, condition of edema, and other clinical manifestations.

a. Combination of wind and water.

Clinical manifestations: Edema often begins in eyelids, and then spreads to the four limbs and the entire body. The onset is acute. Edema in the face is pronounced presenting bright complexion. The pitting disappears quickly after the release of the pressure. Other manifestations include scanty and yellow urine or hematuria, fever, aversion to wind, coughing, a thin and white tongue coating, and a superficial pulse.

Analysis: This syndrome is due to invasion of the body surface by external pathogenic wind. Since wind is marked by upward direction and rapid change, and occurs in gusts, edema caused by wind develops rapidly from the eyelids to the other parts of the body. Bright complexion and pitting disappearing soon after the release of pressure are representative signs of edema due to wind invasion. The accumulation of water in the skin and muscles is the cause of scanty and yellow urine. Damp-heat retaining in the lower Jiao injures the vessels, and thereby results in hematuria. Fever, aversion to wind and coughing are the consequences of impaired function of the lung in dispersing and descending due to invasion of the body surface by wind. A thin and white tongue coating, and a superficial pulse are both signs of pathogenic wind.

b. Invasion of the interior of the body by damp-heat.

Clinical manifestations: Mild or indistinct edema, scanty, deep-yellow urine, a red tongue with yellow or yellow and sticky coating, and a rapid pulse.

Analysis: Invasion of damp-heat into the body causes mild or indistinct edema. Downward movement of damp-heat into the urinary bladder explains scanty, deep-yellow urine. Injury of blood vessels by heat leads to hematuria. A red tongue with yellow or yellow and sticky coating, and a rapid pulse are signs of damp-heat.

c. Deficiency of Qi of the lung and spleen.

Clinical manifestations: Indistinct edema or absence of edema, pale complexion, lassitude, sweating, suscept-ability to common cold, a pale tongue with white coating, and a slow and weak pulse.

Analysis: This syndrome is present at the recovery or late stage of the disease, when the body resistance is still weak. Deficiency of the lung and spleen explains pale complexion and sweating. Weakness of the defensive Qi leads to susceptability to common cold. Deficiency of spleen produces damp, and results in lassitude. A pale tongue with white coating, and a slow and weak pulse are both signs of deficiency of Qi and blood due to deficiency of the spleen.

d. Deficiency of the spleen and kidney.

Clinical manifestations: Pale complexion, systemic edema which is even more pronounced in the lower back and abdomen, pitting which stays after the release of pressure. If deficiency of spleen Yang is more pronounced, symptoms also include loose stool, a distending sensation in the epigastrium and abdomen, lassitude and cold limbs. If deficiency of kindey Yang is more pronounced, the accompanying symptoms include soreness and coldness in the lower back and knees, cold limbs, frequent urination with clear urine which is worse at night. In either case, there is a pale and swollen tongue with white coating, and a deep and thready pulse.

Analysis: Deficiency of the spleen implies dysfunction of the spleen in transporting water and damp. Deficiency of kidney Yang does not allow kidney Qi to dominate water metabolism. Overflow of water and damp into the skin and muscles leads to pale complexion and systemic edema. Downward movement of water and damp explains edema more pronounced in the lower back and abdomen. Pitting which stays after the release of pressure is due to accumulation of water and damp in the skin and muscles following deficiency of spleen Yang. Dysfunction of the spleen in transportation and transformation due to deficiency of the spleen causes loose stool and a distending sensation in the epigastrium and abdomen. Deficiency of kidney Yang means weakness of fire of vital gate and thereby gives rise to soreness and coldness in the lower back and knees, and frequent urination with clear urine which is worse at night. A pale and swollen tongue with a white coating, and a thready and weak pulse are both signs of deficiency of both the spleen and kidney.

Treatment

Biao (symptoms and signs) is treated if the disease is of short duration with acute onset. Ben (underlying cause) is treated if the disease is of long duration with slow onset. The treatment of Biao includes dispersing wind, promoting diuresis, and clearing heat. The emphasis in the treatment of Ben is laid on benefiting Qi, consolidating the body surface, invigorating the spleen and tonifying the kidney.

Chinese herbal medicine:

a. Combination of wind and water.

Treatment principle: To disperse wind and promote diuresis.

Recipe: Mahuang Lianqiao Chixiaodou Tang (Decoction of Herba Ephedrae, Fructus Forsythiae and Semen Phaseoli).

Prescription:

5 g of Mahuang (Herba Ephedrae)

10 g of Lianqiao (Fructus Forsythiae)

20 g of Chixiaodou (Semen Phaseoli)

10 g of Chaobaizhu (Rhizoma Atractylodis Macrocephalae, fried)

10 g of Fuling (Poria)

10 g of Zexie (Rhizoma Alismatis)

10 g of Cheqianzi (Semen Plantaginis)

Explanation: This prescription disperses wind, promotes diuresis and relieves swelling. Mahuang disperses wind and causes perspiration. Lianqiao clears heat. Chixiaodou activates blood circulation and promotes diuresis. Baizhu invigorates the spleen and dries out damp. Fuling discharges damp and invigorates the spleen. Zexie and Cheqianzi promote diuresis and relieve edema.

b. Invasion of the interior of the body by damp-heat.

Treatment principle: To clear heat and promote diuresis.

Recipe: Simiao Wan (Pill of Four Wonderful Ingredients).

Prescription:

10 g of Huangbai (Cortex Phellodentri)

10 g of Cangzhu (Rhizoma Atractylodis)

10 g of Niuxi (Radix Achyranthis Bidentatae)

10 g of Chaoyiren (Semen Coicis, fried)

10 g of Lizhicao (Herba Litchi)

10 g of Cheqiancao (Herba Plantaginis)

10 g of Baimaogen (Rhizoma Imperatae)

Explanation: This prescription clears heat and dries out damp. Huangbai clears heat with its bitter and cold quality. Cangzhu is bitter and warm in nature, and dries out damp. Niuxi is characterized by downward movement. Chaoyiren invigorates the spleen and promotes diuresis. Baimaogen clears heat and discharges damp through urine. Lizhicao and Cheqiancao clear heat and promote diuresis.

c. *Deficiency of Qi of the lung and spleen.*

Treatment principle: To invigorate the spleen and benefit Qi.

Recipe: Shen Ling Baizhu San (Powder of Radix Ginseng, Poria and Rhizoma Atractylodis Macrocephalae) combined with Yupingfeng San (Jade Screen Powder).

Prescription:

10 g of Taizishen (Radix Pseudostellariae)

10 g of Chaobaizhu (Rhizoma Atractylodis Macrocephalae, fried)

10 g of Huangqi (Radix Astragali)

10 g of Shanyao (Rhizoma Dioscoreae)

10 g of Fuling (Poria)

10 g of Chaoyiren (Semen Coicis, fried)

Explanation: Shen Ling Baizhu San invigorates the spleen and resolves damp. Yupingfeng San benefits Qi and consolidates the body surface so as to reinforce body resistance and eliminate pathogenic factors. Taizishen, Chaobaizhu and Huangqi invigorate the spleen and benefit Qi. Shanyao, Fuling and Chaoyiren invigorate the spleen and dispel damp through urine.

d. Deficiency of both the spleen and kidney.

Treatment principle: To warm the kidney and invigorate the spleen.

Recipe: Zhenwu Tang (Decoction for Warming the Kidney).

Prescription:

10 g of Shufuzi (Radix Aconiti Praeparata)

10 g of Fuling (Poria)

10 g of Chaobaizhu (Rhizoma Atractylodis Macrocephalae, fried)

10 g of Chaoyiren (Semen Coicis, fried)

10 g of Zexie (Rhizoma Alismatis)

10 g of Cheqianzi (Herba Plantaginis)

2 slices of Shengjiang (Rhizoma Zingiberis Recens)

Explanation: This prescription warms Yang and promotes diuresis. Fuzi warms kidney Yang, and makes Qi to circulate water. Shengjiang warms the stomach and disperses water. Zexie, Cheqianzi, Fuling and Chaoyiren invigorate the spleen and promote diuresis.

Acupuncture treatment:

a. Combination of wind and water.

Treatment principle: To disperse wind and promote diuresis.

Prescription: Sibai (St. 2) 1, Chengjiang (Ren 24) 1, Wenliu (L.I. 7) 1, Hegu (L.I. 4) 1, Fuliu (K. 7) 1, Fengmen (U.B. 12) 1.

Explanation: Fengmen (U.B. 12), Sibai (St. 2) and Chengjiang (Ren 24) disperse wind and relieve edema in the head and face. Wenliu (L.I. 7), Hegu (L.I. 4) and Fuliu (K. 7) cause perspiration in the case of absence of sweating, and check perspiration in the case of excessive sweating. Therefore, this prescription causes perspiration and relieves edema.

b. Invasion of the interior of the body by damp-heat.

Treatment principle: To clear heat and discharge damp through urine.

Prescription: Shuidao (St. 28) 1, Yinlingquan (Sp. 9) 1, Sanyinjiao (Sp. 6) 1, Xingjian (Liv. 2) 1.

Explanation: Shuidao (St. 28), Yinlingquan (Sp. 9) and Sanyinjiao (Sp. 6) invigorate the spleen and discharge damp through urine. Xingjian (Liv. 2), the Ying-Spring Point of the Liver Channel, clears heat in the lower Jiao.

c. Deficiency of Qi of the lung and spleen.

Treatment principle: To invigorate the spleen, benefit Qi and consolidate the body surface.

Prescription: Pishu (U.B. 20) 1, Shenshu (U.B. 23) 1, Mingmen (Du 4) X, Shuifen (Ren 9) X, Shuidao (St. 28) IX, Sanyinjiao (Sp. 6), Taixi (K. 3) 1.

Points according to symptoms and signs:

Loose stool and abdominal distension: Tianshu (St. 25) IX, Qihai (Ren 6) IX.

Frequent urination with clear urine: Quanyuan (Ren 4) IX.

Explanation: Pishu (U.B. 20), Shenshu (U.B. 23), Mingmen (Du 4) and Taixi (K. 3) warm and tonify the spleen and kidney. Shuifen (Ren 9), Shuidao (St. 28) and Sanyinjiao (Sp. 6) invigorate the spleen and promote diuresis.

If symptoms and signs due to invasion of the heart and lung by water and toxins at the late stage of edema occur, points for first aid are then needled such as Neiguan (P. 6) 1, Shenmen (H. 7) 1, Chize (Lu. 5) 1, Zhongwan (Ren 12) 1, Qihai (Ren 6) 1, Shixuan (Extra.) ↓, Renzhong (Ren 26) L, Xuehai (Sp. 10) 1, and Taichong (Liv. 3) L. A combined method must be adopted at the same time.

Other therapies:

Ear acupuncture.

Points: Liver, Spleen, Stomach, Kidney, Subcortex, Urinary Bladder, Abdomen.

Method: Two to three points are needled bilaterally with moderate stimulation once daily.

Discussion

Combination of wind and water and invasion of the interior of the body by damp-heat are mostly of the excess type, and the method of eliminating pathogenic factors is mainly adopted in the treatment. Deficiency of Qi of the lung and spleen and deficiency of both the spleen and kidney are mostly of the deficiency type, and the method of strengthening body resistance or of both strengthening body resistance and eliminating pathogenic factors is mainly adopted in the treatment.

The sick child should rest in bed and reduce exercises. At the early stage of edema, food with high content of sugar, low content of protein and salt or food without salt is recommended. When edema subsides and urine increases in volume, food then increases in amount and in salt content. It is necessary to prevent and treat various infectious diseases in time, because this can prevent or reduce relapse of edema.

12. Nocturnal Enuresis

Nocturnal enuresis, or bed-wetting, often occurs in children under ten. Bed-wetting under three or due to over playing on day time or to excessive drinking before bed time is not pathological. This disease is relatively stubborn, and may make the sick child feel inferior in a prolonged case.

The principal pathogenesis of nocturnal enuresis is congenital deficiency of kidney or deficiency of Qi of the spleen and lung, either of which may impair the function of the urinary bladder in controlling urine. This disease can also be caused by improper care of parents towards the child who has established a bad habit to urine in bed, or by oxyuriasis, which leads to infection of urinary tract.

Differentiation

This disease is mostly caused by deficiency of the kidney, which impairs the function of the urinary bladder in controlling urine, thus presenting a cold syndrome of the deficiency type.

a. Deficiency of kidney Qi.

Clinical manifestations: Bed-wetting at night which is

not found until waking up, pale complexion, retarded intelligence, clear urine increased in volume on day time, possibly cold limbs in a severe case, a pale tongue with thin and white coating, and a deep and thready or deep and slow pulse.

Explanation: This syndrome is due to congenital deficiency of kidney Qi, which does not allow the urinary bladder to control urine. This explains bed-wetting at night and clear urine increased in volume by day. Deficiency of the kidney implies insufficient production of marrow and undernourishment of the brain, and thereby gives rise to retarded intelligence. Yang Qi, in case of deficiency of kidney Yang, fails to warm up the body, and thus produces pale complexion, cold limbs and aversion to cold. A pale tongue with thin and white coating, and a deep and thready pulse, are both signs of a cold syndrome of the deficiency type.

b. Deficiency of Qi of the spleen and lung.

Clinical manifestations: Frequent bed-wetting with scanty urine, pale complexion, lassitude, anorexia, loose stool, a pale tongue, and a slow pulse.

Explanation: Deficiency of Qi of the spleen and lung is often due to poor recuperation after an illness. Deficiency of the spleen means the dysfunction of the spleen in transportation and transformation of body fluid, while deficiency of the lung implies disturbance of the upper source of body fluid. Under this condition, urination fails to be controlled. All this explains frequent bed-wetting with scanty urine. Deficiency of Qi of the spleen and lung also means an insufficient source for producing Qi and blood and inability to transmit food essence to various parts of the body, thus giving rise to pale complexion and lassitude. Impaired function of the spleen may result in retention of damp in the middle Jiao, and subsequently give rise to anorexia and loose stool. A pale tongue and a slow pulse are both signs of deficiency of Qi.

Treatment

Chinese herbal medicine:

a. Deficiency of kidney Qi.

Treatment principle: To warm and tonify kidney Yang and arrest discharge.

Recipe: Jingui Shenqi Wan (Pill for Restoring the Function of the Kidney) combined with Suoquan Wan (Pill for Reducing Urine).

Prescription: Jingui Shenqi Wan and Suoquan Wan, to be taken twice daily, 5 g each time.

Explanation: These two recipes warm the kidney, invigorate the spleen, warm the urinary bladder and check enuresis.

b. Deficiency of Qi of the spleen and lung.

Treatment principle: To invigorate the spleen and benefit Qi.

Recipe: Suoquan Wan (Pill for Reducing Urine) combined with Buzhong Yiqi Tang (Decoction for Tonifying the Middle Jiao and Benefiting Qi).

Prescription: Suoquan Wan and Buzhong Yiqi Wan, to be taken twice daily, 5 g each time.

Explanation: These two recipes tonify the spleen and lung, raise clear Yang, regulate the opening and closing of the urinary bladder, thereby enabling the urinary bladder to control urine.

Acupuncture treatment:

Treatment principle: To tonify the kidney and check discharge. Acupuncture with the reinforcing method and moxibustion is applied.

Prescription: Shenshu (U.B. 23) T, Ciliao (U.B. 32) 1, Guanyuan (Ren 6) IX, Zusanli (St. 36) T, Sanyinjiao (Sp. 6) T.

Points according to symptoms and signs:

Enuresis in dreams: Yintang (Extra.) 1, Shenmen (H. 7) 1.

Explanation: Shenshu (U.B. 23), Ciliao (U.B. 32) and Guanyuan (Ren 6) tonify the kidney and check discharge. Zusanli (St. 36) and Sanyinjiao (Sp. 6) invigorate the spleen and benefit Qi.

Other therapies:

a. Ear acupuncture.

Points: Kidney, Urinary Bladder, Brain Point, Subcortex, Occiput, Area for Enuresis.

Method: Two to three points are selected at one sitting. Rape seeds are implanted.

b. Massage therapy.

Rub with a circular motion Dantian 200 times, rub the abdomen for 20 minutes, and rub Guiwei 30 times with a circular motion. Rub Shenshu (U.B. 23) until the area becomes hot for older children as well. Treatment is given every afternoon.

Discussion

It is necessary to change the habit of urinating in bed. See to it that the child is not very tired during the day time, and does not drink a lot before bed time. Good therapeutic results are expected if Chinese herbal medicine is combined with acupuncture and moxibustion treatment. Pinworm should be dispelled first before acupuncture treatment is given if enuresis is due to pinworm. If prolonged enuresis is due to spina bifida, the prognosis is poor.

Chapter II
Seasonal Diseases

1. The Common Cold

The common cold is one of the most common diseases of children, and is characterized by fever, aversion to cold, nasal obstruction, runny nose, sneezing, coughing and headache. This disease can occur in all four seasons, but more commonly in winter and spring when there is a drastic change in weather, and in children of all ages. The younger the children are, the more the complications there will be. This is the principal characteristic of the common cold of children, which does not appear in adults.

Children are susceptible to common cold, because their Zang-Fu organs are delicate, skin and muscles are thin and loose, and body resistance is weak. The lung and body surface are diseased in the common cold.

Differentiation

Attention is paid to the nature of the invading pathogenic factors in differentiation. There are two types, wind-cold and wind-heat.

a. Wind-cold.

Clinical manifestations: Fever, aversion to cold, absence of sweating, nasal obstruction with clear discharge, sneezing, coughing, itching of the throat, headache, general aching, absence of thirst, absence of inflamed throat, a thin and white tongue coating, a superficial and tense pulse, and a superficial and red capillary vessel of the index finger.

Analysis: Invasion of the body surface by wind-cold leads to the conflict between the pathogenic factors and body resistance, and thereby produces fever and aversion to cold. The closing of the pores is the cause of absence of sweating. Dysfunction of lung Qi in dispersing results in nasal obstruction with clear discharge, and coughing. Since cold has not yet transformed into heat, there is absence of inflamed throat and thirst. A white tongue coating, a superficial and tense pulse, and a superficial and red capillary vessel are all signs of wind-cold.

b. Wind-heat.

Clinical manifestations: High fever, slightly aversion to wind-cold or absence of aversion to wind-cold, mild sweating, nasal obstruction with purulent discharge, sneezing, coughing, thirst, sore throat, a red tongue tip with thin and white or yellowish coating, a superficial and rapid pulse, and a superficial and purple capillary vessel.

Analysis: This syndrome is due to either invasion by external pathogenic wind-heat or transformation of cold into heat. Invasion of the body surface by pathogenic heat leads to high fever. Sore throat is the result of upward disturbance of pathogenic heat. Coughing is due to dysfunction of the lung in descending. A red tongue tip with yellowish coating, a superficial and rapid pulse, and a superficial and purple capillary vessel are all signs of wind-heat.

Treatment

Chinese herbal medicine:

a. Wind-cold.

Treatment principle: To relieve exterior symptoms with pungent and warm herbs.

Recipe: Jing Fang Baidu San (Powder of Herba Schizonepetae and Radix Ledebouriellae for Relieving Toxins).

Prescription:

5 g of Jingjie (Herba Schizonepetae)

5 g of Fangfeng (Radix Ledebouriellae)

3-5 g of Qianghuo (Rhizoma seu Radix Notopterygii)

10 g of Chaihu (Radix Bupleuri)

5 g of Suye (Folium Perillae)

5 g of Qianhu (Radix Peucedani)

10 g of Zhiqiao (Fructus Aurantii)

5 g of Gancao (Radix Glycyrrhizae)

5 g of Jiegeng (Radix Platycodi)

Explanation: This prescription relieves the exterior symptoms with pungent and warm herbs, eliminates wind and disperses cold. Jingjie, Fangfeng and Qianhu disperse wind-cold. Suye and Qianhu promote the lung's function in dispersing and relieve exterior symptoms. Zhiqiao, Jiegeng and Gancao relax the chest and dispel phlegm. Chaihu clears heat.

b. Wind-heat.

Treatment principle: To relieve exterior symptoms with pungent and cool herbs.

Recipe: Yinqiao San (Powder of Flos Lonicerae and Fructus Forsythiae) or Sang Ju Yin (Decoction of Folium Mori and Flos Chrysanthemi).

Prescription:

If fever is more pronounced, then:

10 g of Lianqiao (Fructus Forsythiae)

10 g of Yinhua (Flos Lonicerae)

10 g of Douchi (Semen Sojae Praeparatum)

5 g of Bohe (Herb Menthae)

10 g of Niubangzi (Fructus Arctii)

5 g of Jingjie (Herba Schizonepetae)

10 g of Chaihu (Radix Bupleuri)

If coughing is more pronounced, then:

10 g of Sangye (Folium Mori)

10 g of Juhua (Flos Chrysanthemi)

5 g of Gancao (Radix Glycyrrhizae)

5 g of Jiegeng (Radix Platycodi)

5 g of Bohe (Herba Menthae)

10 g of Xingren (Semen Armeniacae Amarum)

10 g of Suzi (Fructus Perillae)

Explanation: If fever is pronounced, Yin Qiao San relieves exterior symptoms with pungent and cool herbs, clears heat and dispels toxins. If coughing predominates, Sang Ju Yin promotes the lung's function in dispersing with pungent and cool herbs, resolves phlegm and checks coughing.

c. Complicated syndromes.

(1) In the case of retention of phlegm manifesting as pronounced cough, gurgling with sputum in the throat, a yellowish and thick tongue coating, and a superficial, rolling and rapid pulse, add herbs of resolving phlegm, e.g., 10 g of Yizhihuanghua (Herba seu Radix Solidago Decurrens) and 10 g of Dai Ge San (Powder of Indigo Naturalis and Concha Meretricis seu Cyclinae).

(2) In the case of retention of food with the symptoms of distension and fullness in the epigastrium and abdomen, vomiting with acid smell, foul stool or constipation, a dirty and sticky tongue coating, and a rolling pulse, add herbs of assisting digestion and relieving

139

stagnation, e.g., 10 g of Jiaoshanzha (Fructus Crataegi, burnt), 10 g of Chaoshenqu (Massa Fermentata Medicinalis, fried), and 10 g of Chaolaifuzi (Semen Raphani, fried).

(3) In the case of high fever accompanied by yelling or convulsion (which is relieved as soon as fever subsides), a white or yellowish tongue coating, and a wiry and rapid pulse, add herbs of calming the mind and relieving convulsion, e.g., 5 g of Chanyi (Periostracum Cicadae), 10 g of Gouteng (Ramulus Uncariae cum Uncis), and 10 g of Zhijiangcan (Bombyx Batryticatus, treated); or administer Chinese patent medicines, e.g., Xiaoer Huichun Dan (Regeneration Pill for Children), to be taken two to three pills each time, or Hupo Baolong Wan (Pill of Amber for Holding the Dragon), to be taken 1/2-1 pill each time.

Acupuncture treatment:

a. Wind-cold.

Treatment principle: To eliminate wind and relieve the exterior symptoms.

Prescription: Fengmen (U.B. 12) 1, Feishu (U.B. 13) 1, Quchi (L.I. 11) 1, Hegu (L.I. 4) 1.

Points according to symptoms and signs:

Fever: Dazhui (Du 14) L.

Nasal obstruction with discharge: Yingxiang (L.I. 20) 1.

Headache: Taiyang (Extra.) 1.

Explanation: Fengmeng (U.B. 12) and Feishu (U.B. 13) eliminate wind and cold. Quchi (L.I. 11) and Hegu (L.I. 4) relieve the exterior symptoms and clear heat.

b. Wind-heat.

Treatment principle: To clear heat and relieve the exterior symptoms.

Prescription: Dazhui (Du 14) 1, Quchi (L.I. 11) L, Hegu (L.I. 4) 1, Fengmen (U.B. 12) 1, Feishu (U.B. 13) 1.

Points according to symptoms and signs:

Nasal obstruction with discharge: Yingxiang (L.I. 20) 1.

Sore throat: Yuji (Lu. 10) 1, and Shaoshang (Lu. 11), to be pricked with the three-edged needle to cause bleeding.

Explanation: Dazhui (Du 14), Hegu (L.I. 4) and Quchi (L.I. 11) clear heat and relieve the exterior symptoms. Fengmen (U.B. 12) and Feishu (U.B. 13) promote the lung's function in dispersing and eliminate wind.

c. Complicated syndromes.

(1) Retention of phlegm: Chize (Lu. 5) 1, Fenglong (St. 40) 1.

(2) Retention of food: Zhongwan (Ren 12) 1, Tianshu (St. 25) 1, Qihai (Ren 6) 1, Zusanli (St. 36) 1.

(3) Convulsion: Yintang (Extra.) 1, Shenmen (H. 7) 1, Yanglingquan (G.B. 34) 1, Taichong (Liv. 3) 1.

Other therapies:

Ear acupuncture.

Points: Lung, Trachea, Internal Nose, Ear Apex, Stomach, Spleen, Sanjiao.

Method: Two to three points are chosen bilaterally to be needled with strong stimulation. Needles are retained for 10-20 minutes.

Discussion

High fever and convulsion are likely to occur one to two days after the onset of the common cold in babies and young children; but they rarely occur several times continuously, and convulsion stops as soon as fever subsides.

The sick child should drink plenty of water and eat

food which is easily digestible. Normally, the child should do certain outdoor exercises so as to build up health, and be exposed to the sunshine as much as possible in order to strengthen body resistance.

The early stage of certain acute infectious diseases may have similar symptoms and signs to common cold. It is necessary to make a clear differentiation so as to avoid incorrect diagnosis.

2. Measles

Measles is an acute infectious disease of children marked by fever and small red spots that cover the whole body three days after fever occurs. This disease may occur in all four seasons, but more commonly in winter and spring, and spread among children, especially those between one and five years of age.

Measles is caused by invasion of the Lung and Spleen channels by seasonal pathogenic factors and measles toxins. Other internal organs may also be affected. Proper nursing, correct treatment and full eruption of skin rashes are the conditions for rapid recovery. However, weak body constitution or improper nursing can cause complications. Pneumonia is the most commonly seen complication, which may threaten the child's life.

In China, children have inoculations against measles. The occasional cases of measles present mild symptoms and signs.

Differentiation

Favourable and reverse syndromes should be differentiated first. The former is marked by outward eruption, while the latter is characterized by inward trans-

Differentiation of Favourable and Reverse Syndromes of Measles

		Favourable syndromes		Reverse syndromes
Stage	Before rash appears	Rash appears	Rash fades	Fever is too high or not high enough. High fever does not abate at the last stage.
Fever	Chills and fever.	Continuous fever.	Fever subsides.	
Cough	Mild.	Aggravation.	Less pronounced.	Persistent severe cough, shortness of breath, ala nasi trembling.
Mental state	Normal.	Restlessness.	Normal.	Restlessness, mental cloudiness, delirium.
Sweating	Mild.	Mild.	Mild.	Absence of sweating, dry and heat sensation of the skin, or profuse sweating and cold limbs.

		Favourable syndromes	Reverse syndromes
Skin eruption	Order	Hairlines behind ear, neck, face, back, chest, four limbs, and nose, hands and feet.	Delayed eruption or untimely fading of rash.
	Distribution	Even.	Sparse and indistinct, or dense. and joining up into larger areas, absence of rashes in the face and nose in severe cases.
	Colour	Bright red and moist.	Dark-pale or dark-purple.

144

mission.

a. Favourable syndromes.

(1) Before the rash appears.

Clinical manifestations: Fever with absence of sweating, cough, runny nose, sneezing, redness of the eyes, watery eyes, loose stool, a red tongue with thin and white or slightly yellow coating, and a superficial pulse.

Analysis: Invasion of the lung by measles toxins at the early stage creates fever with absence of sweating. Dysfunction of the lung in descending causes cough. Upward disturbance of measles toxins leads to red and watery eyes. The above-described tongue and pulse are signs of exterior heat syndromes.

(2) The rash appears.

Clinical manifestations: High fever, severe cough, coarse breathing, increased number of thorny and dark-red raised rashes starting first behind the ear then spreading to the head, face, back, chest and four limbs, thirst with desire to drink, a red tongue with yellow and thick or yellow and coarse coating, and a surging and rapid pulse.

Analysis: Retention of measles toxins in the lung and stomach is the cause of high fever and severe cough. The outward movement of toxins leads to distinct skin rashes. A red tongue with yellow and thick or yellow and coarse coating, and a surging and rapid pulse are both signs of heat toxins.

(3) The rash fades.

Clinical manifestations: Both fever and rashes gradually diminish. Cough reduces with little sputum. Both appetite and spirit improve. Thirst is still present. The tongue is red with thin and clean coating and lack of moisture. The pulse is thready and rapid.

Analysis: This stage sees the full eruption of measles toxins from the body surface and gradual recuperation of the body. However, pathogenic heat has already injured Yin of the lung and stomach, thereby manifesting as dry cough with little sputum, thirst, a red tongue with scanty coating and moisture, and a thready and rapid pulse.

b. *Reverse syndrome.*

A reverse syndrome presents grave pathological conditions, and often occurs when the rash appears. Clinically, this syndrome manifests as too high temperature, or fever not high enough, or persistent high fever when rash fades; delayed eruption of skin rashes, or untimely diminishing of skin rashes, or dark-purple densely-distributed rashes.

(1) Blockage of the lung by measles toxins.

Clinical manifestations: High fever, restlessness, cough, shortness of breath, ala nasi trembling, blueish-grey complexion, absence of tears and nasal discharge, dark-purple or indistinct skin rashes, cyanosis of lips, thirst, a red tongue with thin and yellow or yellow and coarse coating, and a rolling and rapid pulse.

Analysis: This syndrome is due to hyperactivity of measles toxins or to complication with pathogenic wind-heat. Blockage of the lung by measles toxins and pathogenic heat makes the symptoms and signs pronounced.

(2) Invasion of the throat by measles toxins.

Clinical manifestations: High fever continues. Skin rashes fade as soon as they appear; or they are densely-distributed and dark-purple in colour. The voice is hoarse. In severe cases, there appear intolerable asthmatic breathing and wheezing, restlessness, and a blueish-grey complexion. A red tongue with yellow and thick coating, and a rolling and rapid pulse are also present.

Analysis: This syndrome is due to disturbance of the throat by measles toxins and pathogenic fire mixed with phlegm. Blockage of the air passage gives rise to a series of throat problems, including suffocation due to throat obstruction in a severe case. This syndrome is often complicated with pneumonia.

(3) Sinking of measles toxins.

Clinical manifestations: High fever, restlessness, delirium, densely-distributed skin rashes which coalesce, petechiae which don't fade on pressure, possibly epistaxis or coma or convulsion in a severe case, a deep-red tongue with yellow coating, and a wiry and rapid pulse.

Analysis: This syndrome is due to invasion of the Ying (nutrient) and Xue (blood) systems and the pericardium by measles toxins and pathogenic heat, and to stirring of liver wind.

Treatment

Chinese herbal medicine:

a. Favourable syndromes.

(1) Before the rash appears.

Treatment principle: To relieve the exterior symptoms and bring the rash out.

Recipe: Yinqiao San (Powder of Flos Lonicerae and Fructus Forsythiae).

Prescription:

10 g of Lianqiao (Fructus Forsythiae)

10 g of Yinhua (Flos Lonicerae)

5 g of Gancao (Radix Glycyrrhizae)

5 g of Jiegeng (Radix Platycodi)

10 g of Niubangzi (Fructus Arctii)

5 g of Jingjie (Herba Schizonepetae)

5 g of Chanyi (Periostracum Cicadae)

Explanation: This prescription relieves exterior symptoms with pungent and cool herbs so as to bring the rash out. Chanyi helps bring the rash out. Lianqiao and Yinhua clear heat and relieve toxins. Gancao and Jiegeng ease the throat and dispel phlegm. Niubangzi and Jingjie relieve the exterior symptoms and bring the rash out.

(2) The rash appears.

Treatment principle: To clear heat and bring the rash out.

Recipe: Qingjie Toubiao Tang (Decoction for Clearing Heat, Relieving Toxins and Bringing the Rash Out).

Prescription:

10 g of Lianqiao (Fructus Forsythiae)

10 g of Yinhua (Flos Lonicerae)

10 g of Huangqin (Radix Scutellariae)

5 g of Chanyi (Periostracum Cicadae)

10 g of Gegen (Radix Puerariae)

10 g of Zicao (Radix Arnebiae seu Lithospermi)

Explanation: This syndrome is present at the peak stage of measles when measles toxins are transmitted outward from the interior of the body. The symptoms and signs due to heat toxins are pronounced at this stage. The emphasis in the treatment is on bringing the rash out and relieving heat toxins. Lianqiao, Yinhua and Huangqin clear heat and relieve toxins. Chanyi and Gegen relieve exterior symptoms and bring the rash out. Zicao clear heat, cools blood, relieves toxins and brings the rash out.

(3) The rash fades.

Treatment principle: To nourish Yin and clear heat of the lung.

Recipe: Shashen Maidong Tang (Decoction of Radix Glehniae and Radix Ophiopogonis).

Prescription:

10 g of Beishashen (Radix Glehniae)

10 g of Maidong (Radix Ophiopogonis)

10 g of Tianhuafen (Radix Trichosanthis)

10 g of Yuzhu (Rhizoma Polygonati Odorati)

10 g of Sangye (Folium Mori)

10 g of Chaobiandou (Semen Dolichoris Album, fried)

5 g of Gancao (Radix Glycyrrhizae)

Explanation: This prescription clears heat, nourishes Yin of the lung and stomach and produces fluid. This effect is achieved with sweet and cold herbs. Beishashen, Maidong, Huafen and Yuzhu nourish Yin fluid of the lung and stomach. Biandou and Gancao pacify and nourish stomach Qi. Sangye clears and brings out pathogenic heat.

b. Reverse syndrome.

(1) Blockage of the lung by measles toxins.

Treatment principle: To clear heat, relieve toxins, promote the lung's function in dispersing and to resolve phlegm.

Recipe: Ma Xing Shi Gan Tang (Decoction of Herba Ephedrae, Semen Armeniacae Amarum, Gypsum Fibrosum and Radix Glycyrrhizae).

Prescription:

5 g of Mahuang (Herba Ephedrae)

10 g of Xingren (Semen Armeniacae Amarum)

30 g of Shigao (Gypsum Fibrosum)

5 g of Gancao (Radix Glycyrrhizae)

10 g of Yuxingcao (Herba Houttuyniae)

10 g of Huangqin (Radix Scutellariae)

Explanation: This prescription is commonly used in the treatment of pneumonia. Since there is hyperactivity of heat toxins, Yuxingcao and Huangqin are prescribed to clear heat and relieve toxins.

(2) Invasion of the throat by measles toxins.

Treatment principle: To clear heat, dispel toxins, ease the throat and relieve swelling.

Recipe: Qingyan Xiatan Wan (Pill for Clearing Heat in the Throat and Dispelling Phlegm).

Prescription:

10 g of Xuanshen (Radix Scrophulariae)
10 g of Niubangzi (Fructus Arctii)
5 g of Gancao (Radix Glycyrrhizae)
5 g of Jiegeng (Radix Platycodi)
10 g of Yinhua (Flos Lonicerae)
5 g of Chuanbeimu (Bulbus Fritillariae Cirrhosae)
10 g of Shandougen (Radix Sophorae Subprostratae)
10 g of Gualou (Fructus Trichosanthis)

Explanation: This prescription clears heat, dispels toxins, eases the throat and relieves swelling. To strengthen the effect of dispelling toxins and easing the throat, administer Liushen Wan (Pill of Six Ingredients with Magical Effects) two to three times daily, one pill for each year of age, each time with the total dosage not exceeding ten pills.

(3) Sinking of measles toxins.

Treatment principle: To clear heat, relieve toxins, calm wind and promote mental resuscitation.

Recipe: Lingjiao Gouteng Tang (Decoction of Cornu Antolopis and Ramulus Uncariae cum Uncis), Niuhuang Qingxin Wan (Calculus Bovis Pill for Clearing Heat in the Heart).

Prescription:

2 g of Lingyangjiao (Corni Antelopis), to be ground with water and taken separately

10 g of Gouteng (Ramulus Uncariae cum Uncis)

5 g of Chuanbeimu (Bulbus Fritillariae Cirrhosae)

10 g of Xianshengdi (Radix Rehmanniae, fresh)

10 g of Danpi (Cortex Moutan Radicis)

10 g of Baishao (Radix Paeoniae Alba)

5 g of Gancao (Radix Glycyrrhizae)

10 g of Yujin (Radix Curcumae)

5 g of Changpu (Rhizoma Acori Graminei)

Also administer Niuhuang Qingxin Wan twice daily, half a pill each time.

Explanation: Lingyangjiao and Gouteng cool the liver and calm wind. Chuanbeimu resolves phlegm. Xianshengdi, Danpi, Baishao and Gancao cool blood, clear heat and nourish the tendons and channels. Changpu and Yujin are both aromatics and promote mental resuscitation. Niuhuang Qingxin Wan clears heat in the heart and relieves toxins.

Discussion

There is a saying in the treatment of measles, "The rash should be brought out first. Once the rash fully appears and toxins are relieved, the prognosis is good." Therefore, it is necessary to keep the pores open and cause constant sweating mildly in order to dispel measles toxins. Measles due to hyperactivity of heat toxins often presents a reverse syndrome, and is likely to be complicated with pneumonia. The method of causing full eruption should be combined with the method of relieving heat and toxins in the treatment at that time, no matter whether the rashes have all been brought out or not.

In summary, the etiological factor of measles is measles toxins, which is characterized by outward movement from the interior of the body. The method to bring the rash out and relieve heat and toxins should be adopted in the entire process of treatment.

The sick child should keep clean the mouth, nose and eyes; eat simple and less salty food which is easily digestible, preferably fluid or half fluid diet. The bedroom should be well ventilated. But the sick child should avoid direct exposure to wind and cold as well as strong light.

The sick child should be isolated until the fifth day after the rash appears, or the tenth day after the rash appears if pneumonia is complicated.

3. Rubella

Rubella is a mild infectious disease marked by mild fever, cough, and sand-sized and light-red skin rashes which appear and fade quickly. There is no desquamation nor skin rash mark after the rash fades. This disease often occurs in winter and spring in children under five years of age with quick recovery and good prognosis. However, if a woman in her third month of pregnancy suffers from rubella, the fetus may possibly be congenitally deformed.

This disease is due to invasion of the lung by external wind-heat via the mouth and nose. Since the invading pathogenic factors are usually mild, only the lung is affected in this disease. The lung connects with the skin and hair. Full eruption of skin rashes brings out pathogenic heat, thereby resolving the disease.

Differentiation

Invasion of the lung and the Wei (defence) system by wind-heat is a general syndrome. Occasionally, the pathogenic factor invades the Qi (vital energy) and Ying (nutrient) systems if heat toxins are hyperactive.

Clinical manifestations: Mild fever (generally 38°C, and over 39°C in a few cases) or aversion to wind, sneezing, runny nose, mild cough, less pronounced restlessness, slightly raised light-red skin rashes, a slightly red tongue with thin and white coating, and a superficial and rapid pulse.

Analysis: Invasion of the lung and the Wei system by external pathogenic wind-heat leads to fever, aversion to wind, cough, sneezing and runny nose. Outward movement of pathogenic wind-heat from the interior of the body creates sparsely distributed and light-red skin rashes. A slightly red tongue with thin and white coating, and a superficial and rapid pulse, are both signs of wind-heat at the body surface.

Treatment

Generally speaking, this disease is treated as exposure to wind-heat, since the symptoms and signs are mild. But a small number of cases may present hyperactivity of heat toxins, and herbs for clearing heat and relieving toxins should be prescribed in a large dosage in such cases.

Chinese herbal medicine:

Treatment principle: To eliminate wind and clear heat.

Recipe: Yinqiao San (Powder of Flos Lonicerae and Fructus Forsythiae).

Prescription:

10 g of Lianqiao (Fructus Forsythiae)

10 g of Yinhua (Flos Lonicerae)

10 g of Niubangzi (Fructus Arctii)
5 g of Jingjie (Herba Schizonepetae)
5 g of Bohe (Herba Menthae)
10 g of Douchi (Semen Sojae Praeparatum)
5 g of Gancao (Radix Glycyrrhizae)
5 g of Jiegeng (Radix Platycodi)

Explanation: This prescription relieves the exterior symptoms with pungent and cool herbs and brings the rash out. Yinhua and Lianqiao clear heat and relieve toxins. Niubangzi, Jingjie, Bohe and Douchi relieve the exterior symptoms and bring the rash out. Gancao and Jiegeng ease the throat and dispel phlegm.

Fever is not high, since the pathogenic factor invades the lung and the Wei (defence) system. If high fever is persistent due to inward transmission of pathogenic heat although the rash has appeared, administer Xiaoer Huichun Dan (Regeneration Pill for Children) two to three times daily, two to three pills each time to prevent convulsion due to high fever.

Discussion

Rubella is due to exposure to wind-heat, and is characterized by mild pathological conditions and a slim chance of transmission and transformation. It is necessary to differentiate rubella from other infectious diseases with skin rashes such as measles, roseola infantum and scarlet fever.

The sick child should be isolated until the fifth day after the occurrence of skin rashes.

4. Scarlet Fever

Scarlet fever is an acute infectious disease marked by

fever, swelling, pain and erosion of the throat, and diffuse bright red skin rashes all over the body. This disease is epidemic in winter and spring. Children between two and eight years of age are likely to be affected.

Scarlet fever is due to invasion of the lung and stomach by external heat toxins via the mouth and nose. Since the throat is the gateway of the lung and stomach, disturbance of the throat by heat toxins leads to redness, swelling, pain and erosion of the throat. Outward disturbance of the muscular surface by heat toxins gives rise to bright red skin eruptions, which may join up into larger areas in severe cases. If heat toxins consume heart Yin and deprive the heart of nourishment, palpitation and pulse with missed beats will occur. If the residual toxins flow into the kidney, the function of the kidney in dominating water metabolism will be impaired. As a result, edema will ensue.

Differentiation

Measles, rubella, roseola infantum and scarlet fever are all infectious diseases with skin eruptions. Attention should be paid to the differentiation of these four diseases.

Fever, sweating, and red and moist skin eruptions suggest outward movement of pathogenic factors, while high fever, absence of sweating, indistinct skin eruptions or purple eruptions mixed with petechiae indicate inward transmission of heat toxins.

a. Invasion of the lung and the Wei (defence) system by the pathogenic factor.

Clinical manifestations: Fever, possibly aversion to cold; then high fever, thirst, headache, cough, sore throat, flushed skin, indistinct bright-red skin eruptions,

Differentiation of Measles, Rubella, Roseola Infantum and Scarlet Fever

	Relation between fever and skin eruptions	Symptoms and signs at the early stage	Characteristics of skin eruptions	Specific signs	Restoration stage
Measles	Skin eruptions occur three to four days after the onset of fever. Fever becomes even higher when rash appears.	Fever, cough, runny nose, watery eyes.	Dark-red maculopapules between which there is normal skin. It takes three days to bring out all eruptions, which occur in a definite order.	Measles, mucous patches.	Furfuraceous desquamation and pigmentation.
Rubella	Skin eruptions occur 1/2–1 day after the onset of fever.	Fever, cough, runny nose, enlarged lymph nodes behind the ear and in the occipital region.	Light-red maculopapules which occur first on the face, then spread rapidly throughout the body in 24 hours, and which are smaller than measles.	None.	No desquamation, or pigmentation.

Roseola infantum	Fever lasts three to four days, and skin eruptions occur when fever subsides.	Sudden high fever. Other symptoms are not severe.	Rosy maculopapules, which are smaller than measles, and may cover the entire body in 24 hours in an indefinite order.	None.	No desqaumation or pigmentation.
Scarlet fever	Skin eruptions occur 1/2-1 day after the onset of fever.	Fever, redness, pain, swelling, and erosion of throat.	Bright-red and densely distributed spots, which coalesce and occur first on the neck, chest and armpit, then spread to entire body in two to three days. Flushed face on which there is no rash.	A pale circle around mouth, red and thorny tongue, thread-like rash in skin creases.	Possibly desquamation, but no pigmentation.

a red tongue with thin and white coating, and a super-ficial and rapid pulse.

Analysis: Invasion of the lung and the Wei system by heat toxins at the early stage impairs the lung's function in dispersing, thereby giving rise to exterior symptoms. Disturbance of the throat by heat toxins leads to sore throat. Indistinct skin eruptions suggest the beginning of outward movement of heat toxins.

b. *Invasion of the Qi (vital energy) and Ying (nutrient) systems by toxins.*

Clinical manifestations: High fever, flushed face, thirst with desire to drink, restlessness, swelling, pain and erosion of the throat, densely distributed and bright-red or purple skin eruptions, dry stool, scanty and deep-yellow urine, a deep-red or thorny tongue with yellow and coarse coating, and a rapid and forceful pulse.

Analysis: This syndrome is due to transformation of heat toxins into fire, which invades the interior of the body and gives rise to excessive internal heat. Heat toxins disturb the throat along the channels, while toxic fire invades the Qi and Ying systems, and gives rise to skin eruptions which densely cover the entire body.

c. *Consumption of Yin when rash fades.*

Clinical manifestations: Gradual diminishing of high fever and skin eruptions, dry skin with desquamation, reduced sore throat, thirst, dryness of lips, dry cough, a red tongue with scanty moisture, and a thready and rapid pulse.

Analysis: This syndrome is present at the restoration stage of the disease when the rash fades and fever subsides. However, heat toxins have turned into fire, which consumes Yin fluid. This explains signs of consumption of Yin of the lung and stomach such as dryness in the mouth and lips, a red tongue with scanty moisture, and dry skin with desquamation.

Treatment

Chinese herbal medicine:

a. Invasion of the lung and Wei (defence) system by the pathogenic factor.

Treatment principle: To promote the lung's function in dispersing and bring the rash out with pungent and cool herbs, clear heat and ease the throat.

Recipe: Yinqiao San (Powder of Flos Lonicerae and Fructus Forsythiae).

Prescription:

10 g of Lianqiao (Fructus Forsythiae)

10 g of Yinhua (Flos Lonicerae)

10 g of Niubangzi (Fructus Arctii)

5 g of Bohe (Herba Menthae)

10 g of Douchi (Semen Sojae Praeparatum)

5 g of Gancao (Radix Glycyrrhizae)

5 g of Jiegeng (Radix Platycodi)

5 g of Chanyi (Periostracum Cicadae)

10 g of Gegen (Radix Pueraiae)

Explanation: This prescription is used at the initial stage of scarlet fever when the pathogenic factor is located at the body surface, or when the rash has started appearing, but has not completely appeared. Lianqiao and Yinhua clear heat and relieve the exterior symptoms. Gegen, Douchi, Chanyi and Bohe relieve exterior symptoms and cause sweating. Gancao and Jiegeng ease the throat. Niubangzi eliminates wind and clears heat. All the herbs combine to dispel the pathogenic factors by sweating and eliminate toxins by bringing out the rashes.

b. Invasion of the Qi and Ying systems by toxins.

Treatment principle: To clear heat in the Qi system, cool the Ying system, reduce fire and relieve toxins.

Recipe: Liangying Qingqi Tang (Decoction for Cooling the Ying System and Clearing Heat in the Qi System).

Prescription:

2 g of Xijiao (Cornu Rhinoceri), to be ground with water and taken separately

10 g of Shengdi (Radix Rehmanniae)

10 g of Danpi (Cortex Moutan Radicis)

10 g of Lianqiao (Fructus Forsythiae)

30 g of Shigao (Gypsum Fibrosum)

10 g of Chaoshanzhi (Fructus Gardeniae, fried)

3 g of Huanglian (Rhizoma Coptidis)

5 g of Gancao (Radix Glycyrrhizae)

10 g of Xuanshen (Radix Scrophulariae)

Explanation: This prescription is used when the rash has densely appeared and there is vigorous heat in the Qi and Ying systems. Xijiao (or buffalo horn, to be used ten times more in dosage), Shengdi and Danpi cool the Ying system and clear heat. Lianqiao, Shigao, Huanglian and Gancao dispel the pathogenic factor from the Qi system. Xuanshen nourishes Yin and clears heat. All the herbs combine to clear heat, relieve toxins, cool the Ying system and produce body fluid.

c. Consumption of Yin when rash fades.

Treatment principle: To nourish Yin, produce body fluid, clear heat and moisten the throat.

Recipe: Shashen Maidong Tang (Decoction of Radix Glehniae and Radix Ophiopogonis).

Prescription:

10 g of Beishashen (Radix Glehniae)

10 g of Maidong (Radix Ophiopogonis)

10 g of Yuzhu (Rhizoma Polygonati Odorati)
10 g of Tianhuafen (Radix Trichosanthis)
10 g of Shihu (Herba Dendrobii)
5 g of Gancao (Radix Glycyrrhizae)
10 g of Sangye (Folium Mori)

Explanation: This prescription is applicable to consumption of Yin of the lung and stomach when desquamation occurs after the rash has completely appeared. Shashen and Maidong clear heat and nourish the lung and stomach. Yuzhu, Shihu and Huafen produce body fluid and relieve thirst. Gancao benefits Qi and tonifies the middle Jiao. Sangye disperses the residual pathogenic factor. All the herbs combine to clear heat and nourish the lung and stomach, promote body fluid and relieve dryness.

Acupuncture treatment:

Prescription: Jinjin (Extra.), Yuyue (Extra.), Dazhui (Du 14), Fengchi (G.B. 20), Sanyinjiao (Sp. 6).

Method: Needling with the reducing method once daily.

Discussion

Scarlet fever is due to invasion by heat toxins. Therefore, the principal method of treatment should be to eliminate heat toxins. Medical scholars of all ages advocate three taboos in the treatment, namely, forbidding the use of pungent and warm herbs to relieve exterior symptoms, forbidding the prescription of cold and bitter herbs too early, and forbidding the use of purgatives to dispel heat downward. Clinical practice has revealed these statements significant. The reason is that to cause drastic sweating is likely to consume body fluid; too early application of bitter and cold herbs inhibits the pathogenic factor from being dispelled; and improper application of purgatives causes sinking of the pathogenic factor to the deeper areas.

The sick child should rest at a quiet place, be given sufficient nourishment and water, keep the skin and mouth clean in order to prevent complications. The sick child should also be isolated for at least seven days, and then urine tested and heart examined in the first month after the recovery.

5. Chickenpox

Chickenpox is a common acute infectious disease of children, and is marked by fever, batches of papules and vesicles, and scabs. This disease is highly epidemic in nurseries and kindergartens in all four seasons, especially in autumn and winter, among children of three to four years old.

This disease is due to invasion by external seasonal pathogenic factors complicated with retention of damp-heat in the interior of the body, and principally involves the Lung and Spleen channels. Outward movement of invading seasonal pathogenic factors brings about vesicles on the body surface. Red and moist vesicles with clear fluid in the centre suggests full eruption of the pathogenic factors on the exterior of the body. Large-sized, densely distributed, and dark-purplish skin eruptions accompanied by high fever, restlessness, thirst and flushed face indicate invasion of the Xue (blood) system by heat toxins.

Differentiation

Generally, the Wei (defence) and Qi (vital energy) systems are diseased in chickenpox. Heat toxins rarely invade the Ying (nutrient) and Xue (blood) systems. The former presents mild pathological conditions, while the latter is severe.

a. Wind-heat (*mild syndrome*).

Clinical manifestations: Mild fever, headache, nasal obstruction with discharge, cough, sneezing, red and moist skin eruptions with clear fluid in the centre, a slightly red tongue with thin and white coating, and a superficial and rapid pulse.

Analysis: Mild fever is due to invasion of the Wei and Qi systems by external seasonal pathogenic factors. Skin eruptions with clear fluid in the centre indicate that heat toxins have reached the body surface from the interior of the body. A slightly red tongue with thin and white coating, and a superficial and rapid pulse are both signs of involvement of the body surface in the disease.

b. Heat toxins (*severe syndrome*).

Clinical manifestations: High fever, restlessness, thirst, redness of lips, flushed face, scanty and deep-yellow urine, large-sized, densely distributed, and dark-purple skin eruptions with slightly turbid fluid in the centre; possibly four to five batches of skin eruptions in succession accompanied by blisters or ulcers in the mouth membrane in severe cases; a red tongue with dry and yellow coating, and a rapid, surging and large pulse.

Analysis: Invasion of the Ying and Xue systems by heat toxins leads to high fever, restlessness, flushed face and redness of the lips. Large-sized and densely distributed skin eruptions with scarlet circle at the root and turbid fluid in the centre are due to hyperactivity of toxins. A red tongue with dry and yellow coating, and a surging and rapid pulse are both signs of hyperactivity of heat toxins.

Treatment

Chinese herbal medicine:

a. Wind-heat (mild syndrome).

Treatment principle: To eliminate wind and clear heat.

Recipe: Yinqiao San (Powder of Flos Lonicerae and Fructus Forsythiae).

Prescription:

10 g of Lianqiao (Fructus Forsythiae)
10 g of Yinhua (Flos Lonicerae)
5 g of Jingjie (Herba Schizonepetae)
10 g of Douchi (Semen Sojae Praeparatum)
5 g of Bohe (Herba Menthae)
10 g of Niubangzi (Fructus Arctii)
5 g of Gancao (Radix Glycyrrhizae)
5 g of Jiegeng (Radix Platycodi)

Explanation: This prescription eliminates wind and clears heat with pungent and cool herbs, and relieves toxins. Lianqiao and Yinhua clear heat and relieve toxins, and bring out the pathogenic factors with their pungent and cool properties. Jingjie, Douchi and Bohe relieve the exterior symptoms and dispel pathogenic factors. Niubangzi, Gancao and Jiegeng disperse lung Qi in a mild way.

b. Heat toxins (severe syndrome).

Treatment principle: To clear heat and cool the Ying system.

Recipe: Qingli Jiedu Tang (Decoction for Clearing Heat in the Interior of the Body and Relieving Toxins).

Prescription:

10 g of Huangqin (Radix Scutellariae)
3 g of Huanglian (Rhizoma Coptidis)
30 g of Shigao (Gypsum Fibrosum)

10 g of Shengdi (Rhizoma Rehmannia)

10 g of Danpi (Cortex Moutan Radicis)

Explanation: This prescription clears heat and cools the Ying system, and also relieves toxins. Huangqin and Huanglian clear heat and relieve toxins. Shigao is good at clearing heat from the Qi system. Shengdi and Danpi clear heat and cool blood.

Discussion

Since chickenpox is highly epidemic, the sick child should be isolated immediately until all skin eruptions have dried up and scabs are formed. Simple and less salty food which is easily digestible is recommended. Drinking mung bean soup clears heat and relieves toxins. Don't scratch the skin in order to avoid infection. If blisters break, smear the lesion with 2 percent gentian violet.

6. Mumps

Mumps is an acute infectious disease marked by fever, and swelling and pain in the parotid region. This disease may occur in all four seasons, but it is more epidemic in winter and spring among school-age children.

This disease is due to invasion of the Shaoyang Channel by wind-heat toxins via the mouth and nose. The pathogenic factors may transmit from the Shaoyang to the Jueyin Channel, since these two channels are related both externally and internally. As a result, pain in the lower abdomen or swelling and pain of the testes may occur in a severe case in older children, because these areas are passed through by the Jueyin Channel of Foot. In young children, hyperactive heat toxins may invade the heart and liver, thereby disturbing the mind and stirring wind with the ensuing symptoms of high fever, coma and convulsion.

Differentiation

a. Heat toxins on the exterior of the body.

Clinical manifestations: Mild fever and aversion to cold, swelling and pain of the parotid region on one side or both sides, difficulty in chewing, possibly inflamed throat, a red tongue with thin and white or slightly yellow coating, and a superficial and rapid pulse.

Analysis: This syndrome is present at the early stage of mumps. Invasion of the muscular surface by heat toxins gives rise to fever, aversion to cold and inflamed throat. Swelling of the parotid region is due to invasion of the Shaoyang Channel by heat toxins which cause retarded circulation of Qi and blood in the channel and the parotid region in particular. A red tongue with thin and white coating, and a superficial and rapid pulse are signs of invasion of the exterior part of the body by wind-heat toxins.

b. Retention of heat toxins in the interior.

Clinical manifestations: High fever, headache, thirst with desire to drink, possibly vomiting; swelling and distending pain of the parotid region which feels hard on palpation, and painful on pressure; difficulty in chewing; redness, swelling and pain of the throat; a red tongue with yellow coating, and a rolling and rapid pulse.

Analysis: This syndrome is due to inward transmission of heat toxins. Since heat toxins are hyperactive, both systemic and regional symptoms and signs are pronounced, and complications are likely to occur.

Treatment

Combination of oral administration of Chinese herbal decoction with external application of drugs or acupuncture is conducive to relief of swelling.

a. Heat toxins on the exterior of the body.

Treatment principle: To eliminate wind, clear heat, disperse the mass and relieve swelling.

Recipe: Yinqiao San (Powder of Flos Lonicerae and Fructus Forsythiae).

Prescription:

10 g of Lianqiao (Fructus Forsythiae)

10 g of Yinhua (Flos Lonicerae)

5 g of Bohe (Herba Menthae)

10 g of Niubangzi (Fructus Arctii)

10 g of Banlangen (Radix Isatidis)

10 g of Xiakucao (Spica Prunellae)

10 g of Zhijiangcan (Bombyx Batryticatus, treated)

Explanation: Yinhua and Lianqiao clear heat and relieve toxins. Niubangzi and Bohe eliminate wind and clear heat. Banlangen and Xiakucao clear heat, dispel toxins, relieve swelling and soften the hard masses. Zhijiangcan strengthens the effect of eliminating wind, relieving toxins and dispersing the masses.

b. Retention of heat toxins in the interior.

Treatment principle: To clear heat, dispel toxins, soften the hard messes and relieve swelling.

Recipe: Puji Xiaodu Yin (Decoction for General Relief and Dispelling Toxins).

Prescription:

10 g of Huangqin (Radix Scutellariae)

10 g of Lianqiao (Fructus Forsythiae)

10 g of Banlangen (Radix Isatidis)

10 g of Xuanshen (Radix Scrophulariae)

3 g of Mabo (Lasiosphaera seu Calvatia)

10 g of Zhijiangcan (Bombyx Batryticatus, treated)

10 g of Xiakucao (Spica Prunellae)

Explanation: This prescription is applicable to both severe syndrome of retention of heat toxins in the interior and mild syndrome of heat toxins on the exterior of the body. But Huangqin should be removed in the treatment of the mild syndrome of one to two days of duration, because this herb is bitter and cold in nature and thereby it may prevent the pathogenic factor from being dispelled. In this prescription, Huangqin, Lianqiao and Banlangen clear heat and relieve toxins. Xuanshen and Mabo clear heat and ease the throat. Jiangcan and Xiakucao clear heat, remove obstruction in the channels and disperse the masses. If the hard mass in the parotid region persists, add 10 g of Kunbu (Thallus Laminariae seu Eckloniae) and 10 g of Haizao (Sargassum).

External application of drugs to the parotid region and testes is often combined with oral administration of Chinese herbal decoction in the treatment of mumps. If the systemic symptoms are not pronounced and swelling of the parotid region is mild, only external application is adopted. The commonly used drugs for external application include Zijin Ding (Purple Gold Pill), which is also called Yushu Dan (Jade Pivot Pill), and Ruyi Jinhuang San (Golden Yellow Powder for Good Luck). They are mixed evenly with a small amount of green tea fluid and honey and applied to the affected areas.

Acupuncture treatment:

Treatment principle: To eliminate wind, clear heat and disperse the mass.

Prescription: Yifeng (S.J. 17) L, Jiache (St. 6) L, Hegu (L.I. 4) L, Tianrong (S.I. 17) 1.

Points according to symptoms and signs:

Fever: Quchi (L.I. 11) L, Dazhui (Du 14) L.

Swelling and pain of the testes: Xuehai (Sp. 10) 1, Sanyinjiao (Sp. 6) L.

Discussion

Mumps should be differentiated from lymphadenitis in front of the ear and suppurative parotitis. The border of swelling is distinct and there is no redness and swelling of the outlet of the parotid duct in lymphadenitis. Suppurative parotitis often involves one side of the parotid region, and presents redness of the local skin, pronounced tenderness, a water flowing sensation in the case of formation of abscess, and discharge of pus at the outlet of the parotid duct on pressure.

The sick child should be isolated until three to seven days after the relief of swelling of the parotid region.

7. Whooping Cough

Whooping cough is an infectious disease of the respiratory tract marked by paroxysmal gasping coughs and long, noisy indrawing of breath. This disease may occur in all four seasons, but more commonly in winter and spring in children under five years of age. The newborn is also likely to suffer from this disease with critical conditions such as convulsion and suffocation. This disease may last as long as three months.

The early stage of the disease is due to invasion of the lung and the Wei system by seasonal pestilential factor, which makes lung Qi disturb upward and thereby causes cough that is similar to the common cold. If the invading pestilential factor is not dispelled, it turns into fire which condenses fluid into phlegm. The combination of fire and phlegm blocks the air passage and makes the upward dirturbance of lung Qi even worse. As a result, severe gasping coughs follow and will not be relieved until expectoration of sputum. Long-standing cough at the late stage of the disease injures the lung and spleen and causes deficiency of both Qi and Yin, although phlegm and heat have been cleared by then.

Differentiation

a. Invasion of the lung by pathogenic wind (early stage).

Clinical manifestations: The early stage of whooping cough presents similar symptoms and signs to the common cold. The cough is in a heavy voice, worse at night, and aggravates with each passing day. Invasion by wind-cold also manifests as clear and dilute sputum, aversion to cold, a thin and white tongue coating, and a superficial and tense pulse. Invasion by wind-heat also exhibits thick sputum, inflamed throat, a red tongue with thin and yellow coating, and superficial and rapid pulse.

Analysis: Wind may associate itself with either cold or heat in the invasion of the lung and Wei system. Dysfunction of the lung in dispersing and descending is the cause of cough which is worse at night, and aggravates day by day.

b. Retention of phlegm-fire in the lung (stage of gasping cough).

Clinical manifestations: This stage is marked by paroxysmal gasping coughs in strong voice with thick sputum which is difficult to expectorate, noisy indrawing of breath, vomiting and flushed face; possibly bleeding in the eye, gums and nose, or blood-tinged sputum in severe cases; redness, swelling and erosion of glossodesmus in babies; a red tongue with yellow and sticky coating, and a rolling and rapid pulse.

Analysis: The pestilential factor turns into fire, which condenses fluid into phlegm. The combination of phlegm and fire blocks the air passage and disturbs lung Qi. This explains paroxysmal gasping coughs with thick sputum which is difficult to expectorate. Injury of the blood vessels by phlegm fire causes bleeding.

c. Deficiency of both the lung and spleen (recovery stage).

Clinical manifestations: Paroxysmal cough is gradually reduced, and noisy indrawing of breath disappears. Deficiency of lung Yin presents cough in hoarse voice, thirst, a red tongue with scanty coating, and a rapid and weak pulse. Deficiency of spleen Qi manifests as cough in weak and feeble voice, a pale tongue with thin and white coating, and a slow and weak pulse.

Analysis: This syndrome is present at the late stage of whooping cough with deficiency of body resistance which is more pronounced than invading pathogenic factor. Long-standing cough consumes lung Yin and thereby gives rise to cough in hoarse voice and a red tongue. Deficiency of the lung affects the spleen due to long-standing cough, and the result is cough in weak voice and a pale tongue.

Treatment

Since the principal symptom of this disease is gasping cough, which is a sign of phlegm blockage, the method of resolving phlegm and sending perverse Qi downward should be adopted at all stages of treatment.

a. Invasion of the lung by pathogenic wind.

Treatment principle: To promote the lung's function in dispersing and resolve phlegm.

Recipe: Sanao Tang (Decoction of Three Ingredients

for Eliminating Wind-cold) or Sang Ju Yin (Decoction of Folium Mori and Flos Chrysanthemi).

Prescription:

Sanao Tang is applied in the case of wind-cold. The prescription consists of the following:

5 g of Mahuang (Herba Ephedrae)

10 g of Xingren (Semen Armeniacae Amarum)

5 g of Gancao (Radix Glycyrrhizae)

10 g of Zhibaibu (Radix Stemonae, treated)

5 g of Baiqian (Rhizoma Cynanchi Stauntonii)

10 g of Tianzhuzi (Fructus Nandinae Domesticae)

Sang Ju Yin is recommended in the case of wind-heat. The prescription consists of the following:

10 g of Sangye (Folium Mori)

10 g of Juhua (Flos Chrysanthemi)

10 g of Niubangzi (Fructus Arctii)

10 g of Xingren (Semen Armeniacae Amarum)

5 g of Gancao (Radix Glycyrrhizae)

5 g of Jiegeng (Radix Platycodi)

10 g of Dai Ge San (Powder of Indigo Naturalis and Concha Meretricis seu Cyclinae)

Explanation: Sanao Tang is pungent and warm in nature, and effective in promoting the lung's function in dispersing and eliminating cold. The addition of Baibu, Baiqian and Tianzhuzi strengthens the effect of checking cough and resolving phlegm.

Sang Ju Yin is pungent and cool in nature, and is used here mainly for checking cough, although in a mild way it promotes the lung's function in dispersing. The addition of Dai Ge San strengthens the effect of clearing heat and resolving phlegm.

b. Retention of phlegm-fire in the lung.

Treatment principle: To reduce the lung and dispel

phlegm.

Recipe: Sangbaipi Tang (Decoction of Cortex Mori Radicis).

Prescription:

10 g of Sangbaipi (Cortex Mori Radicis)

10 g of Huangqin (Radix Scutellariae)

2 g of Huanglian (Rhizoma Coptidis)

10 g of Chaoshanzi (Fructus Gardeniae, fried)

10 g of Suzi (Fructus Perillae)

10 g of Xingren (Semen Armeniacae Amarum)

5 g of Chuanbeimu (Bulbus Fritillariae Cirrhosae)

10 g of Tinglizi (Semen Lepidii seu Descurainiae)

10 g of Zhibaibu (Radix Stemonae, treated)

10 g of Tianzhuzi (Fructus Nandinae Domesticae)

Explanation: This prescription clears heat, reduces the lung, dispels phlegm and sends perverse Qi downward. Sangbaipi, Tinglizi, Huangqin, Huanglian and Chaoshanzhi clear heat in the lung and reduce the lung. Suzi, Xingren and Chuanbeimu resolve phlegm and send perverse qi downward. Zhibaibu and Tianzhuzi resolve phlegm and check cough.

c. Deficiency of both the lung and spleen.

Treatment principle: To nourish the lung and invigorate the spleen.

Recipe: Renshen Wuweizi Tang (Decoction of Radix Ginseng and Fructus Schisandrae).

Prescription:

10 g of Chaodangshen (Radix Codonopsis Pilosulae, fried)

10 g of Chaobaizhu (Rhizoma Atractylodis Macrocephalae, fried)

10 g of Fuling (Poria)

5 g of Gancao (Radix Glycyrrhizae)

10 g of Maidong (Radix Ophiopogonis)

5 g of Wuweizi (Fructus Schisandrae)

5 g of Chenpi (Pericarpium Citri Reticulatae)

10 g of Fabanxia (Rhizoma Pinelliae, alum treated)

Explanation: This prescription is recommended in the case of deficiency of lung Yin and spleen Qi. Dangshen, Baizhu, Fuling and Gancao invigorate the spleen and benefit Qi. Maidong and Wuweizi moisten the lung and check cough. Chenpi and Fabanxia resolve phlegm.

Acupuncture treatment:

Treatment principle: To clear heat in the lung and resolve phlegm.

Prescription: Chize (Lu. 5) L, Hegu (L.I. 4) L, Fenglong (St. 40) 1, Feishu (U.B. 13) L.

Method: They are needled once daily. Seven sessions comprise a course.

Other therapies:

a. Plum blossom needle is applied to tap the areas within 3-4 cm on both sides of cervical and sacral vertebrae once daily.

b. Cupping.

Apply cupping over Shenzhu (Du 12) once daily.

Discussion

The early and middle stages of whooping cough present syndromes of the excess type, while the late stage is a complicated syndrome between excess and deficiency. Since retention of turbid phlegm blocking the air passage is the main pathogenesis of all three stages of the disease, the method of resolving phlegm, sending perverse Qi downward and circulating lung Qi is always used, in addition to promoting the lung's function in dispersing at the early stage, reducing the lung at the middle stage, and moistening the lung at the late stage.

The sick child should eat simple and less salty food which is easily digestible, and avoid irritation of smoke, dust and strong smells. The sick child must be isolated immediately for four to six weeks.

8. Diphtheria

Diphtheria is an acute infectious disease of the respiratory tract marked by formation of grey-white false membrane over the mucous membrane of the pharynx, larynx and nose, which is accompanied by fever, sore throat, or cough with noisy indrawing of breath. This disease may occur in all four seasons, but it is more epidemic in autumn and winter among children between two and five years of age. The younger the children are, the more severe the pathological conditions will be. Due to constant effort in prevention, the incidence of diphtheria has dropped considerably.

The seasonal pestilential factor of diphtheria directly invades the lung and stomach via the mouth and nose. Since the throat is the gateway of the lung and stomach, upward disturbance of accumulated heat in these organs produces a grey-white false membrane in the throat. The transformation of the invading pestilential factor into fire develops diphtheria from the pharynx to the larynx. Diphtheria of the larynx may also directly result from invasion of the larynx by the pestilential factor. If the pestilential factor is persistent, and the body constitution of the child is weak, the heart or the channels and collaterals can be affected.

Differentiation

a. Diphtheria due to wind-heat.

Clinical manifestations: Mild fever, inflamed, swollen and sore throat, spot-like false membrane in the throat which is hard to remove, difficulty in swallowing, a red tongue tip with thin and white coating, and a superficial and rapid pulse.

Analysis: This syndrome is present at the early stage of diphtheria with mild pathological conditions and involvement of the pharynx. Invasion of the lung and stomach by wind-heat toxins presents similar symptoms and signs to the common cold. The exception is visible false membrane in the throat at the early stage of diphtheria.

b. Diphtheria due to deficiency of Yin.

Clinical manifestations: Inflamed and swollen throat with stripes of grey-white or grey-yellow false membrane, which spreads to the uvula and upper palate in a severe case, dryness of the mouth and throat, fever, cough in a hoarse voice, foul breath, a deep-red tongue with little moisture and thin and yellow coating, and a thready and rapid pulse.

Analysis: This syndrome is due to inward transmission of wind-heat or heat toxins. Disturbance of the throat by heat toxins creates grey-white false membrane, which may spread to the uvula and upper palate. Dry heat consumes Yin and deprives the lung of moisture. This explains dryness of the mouth and throat, and cough in a hoarse voice. Deficiency of Yin fluid with excess of heat toxins is the cause of a deep-red tongue with little moisture and a thready and rapid pulse.

c. Diphtheria due to pestilential factor.

Clinical manifestations: The extreme severe stage of pharyngeal diphtheria presents pronounced sore throat, grey false membrane spreading to and exceeding the tonsils, and swelling of the neck like a cow's. In laryngeal diphtheria, the grey false membrane spreads to the larynx or even to the trachea in a severe case. Other manifestations include cough in a hoarse voice with noisy indrawing of breath, inspiratory dyspnea, restlessness and cyanosis of the lips. In both cases, the tongue is red with yellow and thick coating, and the pulse is rolling and rapid.

Analysis: This syndrome is present at the extreme severe stage of pharyngeal diphtheria or in laryngeal diphtheria due to transformation of pestilential factor into fire. The accumulation of toxins leads to dysharmony of Qi and blood, thereby causing swelling of the neck. Toxic heat condenses fluid into phlegm, which blocks lung Qi and thus gives rise to gurgling with sputum, cough in hoarse voice with noisy indrawing of breath. Obstruction of Qi leads to blood stagnation, which is manifested in cyanosis of the lips or throat obstruction with suffocation in a severe case. A red tongue with yellow coating, and a rolling and rapid pulse are both signs of toxic fire and heat.

Treatment

Generally, the method of nourishing Yin, clearing heat in the lung and relieving toxins is adopted. If there are exterior symptoms, the method of relieving exterior symptoms with pungent and cool herbs is also used. Since the pestilential factor is likely to turn into fire and consume Yin, pungent and warm herbs are not used to relieve the exterior symptoms.

Chinese herbal medicine:

a. Diphtheria due to wind-heat.

Treatment principle: To eliminate wind, clear heat

177

and relieve toxins.

Recipe: Yinqiao San (Powder of Flos Lonicerae and Fructus Forsythiae).

Prescription:

10 g of Lianqiao (Fructus Forsythiae)

10 g of Yinhua (Flos Lonicerae)

5 g of Gancao (Radix Glycyrrhizae)

5 g of Jiegeng (Radix Platycodi)

10 g of Niubangzi (Fructus Arctii)

5 g of Bohe (Herba Menthae)

15 g of Tuniuxi (Radix Achyranthis Asperae)

Explanation: This prescription eliminates wind, relieves the exterior symptoms, clears heat and dispels toxins. Lianqiao and Yinhua clear heat and relieve toxins. Gancao, Jiegeng and Niubangzi ease the throat and dispel toxins. Bohe eliminates wind and clears heat. Tuniuxi dispels heat toxins of diphtheria.

b. Diphtheria due to deficiency of Yin.

Treatment principle: To nourish Yin, clear heat in the lung and relieve toxins.

Recipe: Yangyin Qingfei Tang (Decoction for Nourishing Yin and Clearing Heat in the Lung).

Prescription:

10 g of Shengdi (Radix Rehmanniae)

10 g of Xuanshen (Radix Scrophulariae)

10 g of Maidong (Radix Ophiopogonis)

5 g of Chuanbeimu (Bulbus Fritillariae Cirrhosae)

10 g of Baishao (Radix Paeoniae Alba)

10 g of Danpi (Cortex Moutan Radicis)

10 g of Tuniuxi (Radix Achyranthis Asperae)

5 g of Gancao (Radix Glycyrrhizae)

Explanation: This prescription nourishes Yin, produces moisture, clears fire and relieves toxins. It is not only applicable to this syndrome, but also effective in the treatment of diphtheria as a whole. Shengdi and Xuanshen nourish Yin and produce moisture. Maidong and Chuanbeimu moisten the lung and resolve phlegm. Baishao and Danpi cool blood and reduce fire. Tuniuxi and Gancao clear fire and relieve toxins.

c. *Diphtheria due to pestilential factor.*

Treatment principle: To ease the throat, dispel phlegm and relieve toxins.

Recipe: Shenxian Huoming Yin (Immortal Decoction for Saving Life).

Prescription:

3 g of Longdancao (Radix Gentianae)

3 g of Huanglian (Rhizoma Coptidis)

10 g of Huangqin (Radix Scutellariae)

10 g of Chaoshanzhi (Fructus Gardeniae, fried)

10 g of Huangbai (Cortex Phellodendri)

10 g of Xuanshen (Radix Scrophulariae)

10 g of Shengdi (Radix Rehmanniae)

10 g of Baishao (Radix Paeoniae Alba)

15 g of Tuniuxi (Radix Achyranthis Asperae)

5 g of Gancao (Radix Glycyrrhizae)

Explanation: This prescription nourishes Yin, clears heat, reduces fire and relieves toxins. Longdancao, Huangbai and Chaoshanzhi reduce fire and relieve toxins. Xuanshen, Baishao and Shengdi nourish Yin and clear heat. Tuniuxi and Gancao relieve toxins and ease the throat. Huanglian and Huangqin strengthen the effect of clearing heat and relieving toxins.

Acupuncture treatment:

Treatment principle: To ease the throat and dispel phlegm.

Prescription: Tiantu (Ren 22) 1, Lianquan (Ren 23) 1.

Points according to symptoms and signs:

Excessive phlegm: Fenglong (St. 40) 1.

Cough, shortness of breath and difficulty in swallowing: Shanzhong (Ren 17) 1, Neck-Futu (L.I. 18) 1. '

Sore throat: Hegu (L.I. 4) L, Shaoshang (Lu. 11) ↓.

Discussion

Diphtheria presents many syndromes with critical and complicated symptoms and signs. A correct and immediate treatment should be given. A combined method is usually adopted in the treatment. The sick child should be isolated until two weeks after the relief of all the symptoms and signs including complete disappearance of the grey-white false membrane. Simple and less salty food which is easily digestible and has nutritive value is recommended.

9. Epidemic Encephalitis B

Epidemic encephalitis B is an acute febrile disease of children marked by high fever, convulsion, coma and sudden collapse. This disease occurs in summer and autumn, but more commonly in July, August and September, in children under ten years of age, especially those under five.

This disease is due to invasion of toxic pathogenic factors. Summer heat is often combined with damp in causing disease. Extreme heat produces wind, while excessive wind produces phlegm. That is why this disease presents clinically high fever, coma, convulsion and gurgling with sputum in the throat, which may all transform into each other. Severe cases are likely to leave behind after-effects.

Differentiation

Epidemic encephalitis B is differentiated according to the four stages of Wei (defence), Qi (vital energy), Ying (nutrient) and Xue (blood). Due to abrupt onset of the disease and rapid transmission and transformation, however, it is difficult to clearly distinguish between these four stages. Syndromes of two stages are often present at the same time.

a. Invasion of the Wei (defence) and Qi (vital energy) systems by the pathogenic factor.

Clinical manifestations: Burning sensation of the whole body, absence of sweating, headache, aversion to wind, thirst, vomiting, lethargy or restlessness, neck rigidity, convulsion due to high fever, a red tongue with thin and white or yellow coating, and a superficial and rapid or rolling and rapid pulse.

Analysis: Both the Wei and Qi systems are diseased at the initial stage of the disease. High fever, restlessness, and thirst are symptoms of the Qi stage, while slight aversion to wind is a sign of the Wei stage. A burning sensation of the skin without sweating is not present in the pure syndrome of the Qi stage which presents sweating and thirst. Invasion of the Qi system by the pathogenic factor often involves the Yangming Channel, and thereby impairs the function of the stomach in descending with the result of vomiting. Extreme heat produces wind, and this is why convulsion occurs when there is high fever. The complication of damp is shown in a white, sticky and slightly yellow tongue coating, while excess of heat produces a yellow tongue coating. A superficial and rapid or rolling and rapid pulse is a sign of exterior heat syndrome of the excess type.

b. Invasion of the Qi and Ying systems by pathogenic

factor.

Clinical manifestations: Persistent high fever, mental cloudiness or alternate mental cloudiness and clarity, neck rigidity, convulsion of the four limbs, gurgling with sputum in the throat, constipation, a deep-red tongue with yellow and coarse coating, and a wiry and rapid pulse.

Analysis: Both the Qi and Ying systems are diseased in this extreme stage of the disease. The pathogenic summer heat and heat toxins in the Qi system turn into fire which invades the Ying system. This explains high fever, convulsion and coma. Excessive heat produces phlegm, which blocks the air passage and thereby causes gurgling with sputum in the throat when acted on by internal wind. Excessive heat in the large intestine leads to constipation. A deep-red tongue with yellow and coarse coating, and a wiry and rapid pulse are signs of invasion of the Ying system by extreme heat.

c. Invasion of the Ying and Xue systems by pathogenic factor.

Clinical manifestations: Fever which is more pronounced at night, mental cloudiness, frequent fits of convulsion, dark-grey complexion, possibly hematemesis or even ceasing of respiration temporarily in a severe case, a dark-purple and dry or a rolled and rigid tongue, and a thready and rapid pulse.

Analysis: This syndrome is present at the extreme stage of the disease with critical pathological conditions. Pathogenic summer heat turns into fire, which invades the Xue system and consumes kidney Yin. This explains fever which is more pronounced at night. Since the heart dominates blood and relates to the Ying system, invasion of the Ying system by the pathogenic factor clouds the mind and thus leads to mental cloudiness. Since the liver stores blood, invasion of blood by heat consumes liver Yin and stirs liver wind. The result is frequent fits of convulsion and dark-grey complexion. Excessive heat in the Xue system damages the blood vessels and thereby hematemesis occurs. Blockage of lung Qi leads to dyspnea or ceasing of respiration temporarily. A dark-purple and dry or a rolled and rigid tongue, and a thready and rapid pulse are all signs of consumption of Yin by excessive heat, retention of heat in the Xue system, and Yin deficiency stirring wind.

Treatment

The treatment principle at the acute stage of the disease is to clear heat and preserve body fluid. If damp is pronounced, the method of clearing heat is assisted by the method of resolving damp with aromatics or by the method of dispelling damp via urination with sweet and mild-flavoured herbs. Since high fever is a main symptom, efforts should be made to lower it, which is the key to the recovery of the disease. Convulsion and coma are treated accordingly. When the disease develops to the recovery stage or after-effects occur, acupuncture and massage therapy should be combined with Chinese herbal medicine.

a. Invasion of the Wei and Qi systems by pathogenic factor.

Treatment principle: To relieve the exterior symptoms with pungent and cool herbs, clear heat, and dispel toxins.

Recipe: Xinjia Xiangru Yin (Newly Revised Decoction of Herba Elsholtziae seu Moslae) or Baihu Tang (White Tiger Decoction).

Prescription:

Herbs based on Xinjia Xiangru Yin include:

5 g of Xiangru (Herba Elsholtziae seu Moslae)

5 g of Bohe (Herba Menthae)

10 g of Gegen (Radix Puerariae)

10 g of Douchi (Semen Sojae Praeparatum)

10 g of Lianqiao (Fructus Forsythiae)

10 g of Yinhua (Flos Lonicerae)

10 g of Huoxiang (Herba Agastachis)

10 g of Liuyi San (Powder of Talcum and Raw Radix Glycyrrhizae)

Herbs based on Baihu Tang include:

30 g of Shigao (Gypsum Fibrosum)

5 g of Zhimu (Rhizoma Anemarrhenae)

3 g of Bohe (Herba Menthae)

10 g of Doujuan (Dry Bean Sprouts)

10 g of Lianqiao (Fructus Forsythiae)

10 g of Yinhua (Flos Lonicerae)

10 g of Huangqin (Radix Scutellariae)

5 g of Gancao (Radix Glycyrrhizae)

Explanation: Xinjia Xiangru Yin is applicable to invasion of the Wei (defence) system by pathogenic summer heat, and acts to relieve the exterior symptoms. Xiangru, pungent and warm in nature, relieves the exterior symptoms in summer. Gegen, Bohe and Douchi, all pungent and cool in nature, relieve the exterior symptoms. Lianqiao and Yinhua clear heat and relieve toxins. Huoxiang and Liuyi San resolve turbid damp and dispel damp via urination respectively.

Baihu Tang is recommendable to invasion of the Qi system by pathogenic summer heat, and acts to clear heat in the interior of the body. Shigao, Zhimu and Gancao clear heat and produce body fluid. Lianqiao, Yinhua and Huangqin clear heat and relieve toxins.

Bohe and Doujuan dispel summer heat and damp.

b. Invasion of the Qi and Ying systems by pathogenic factor.

Treatment principle: To clear heat in the Qi and Ying systems, reduce fire and dispel phlegm.

Recipe: Qingwen Baidu Yin (Decoction for Clearing Evil Heat and Relieving Toxins).

Prescription:

30 g of Shigao (Gypsum Fibrosum)

5 g of Zhimu (Rhizoma Anemarrhenae)

5 g of Gancao (Radix Glycyrrhizae)

10 g of Lianqiao (Fructus Forsythiae)

10 g of Shanzhi (Fructus Gardeniae)

3 g of Huanglian (Rhizoma Coptidis)

10 g of Shengdi (Radix Rehmanniae)

10 g of Chishao (Radix Paeoniae Rubra)

10 g of Danpi (Cortex Moutan Radicis)

30 g of Zhuli (Bamboo Juice Obtained with Heating), to be mixed with water and taken separately

Explanation: This prescription clears heat in the Qi system and relieves toxins in the Ying system. Shigao, Zhimu and Gancao clear heat in the Qi system. Lianqiao, Shanzhi and Huanglian reduce fire and relieve toxins. Shengdi, Chishao and Danpi cool the Ying system. Zhuli dispels phlegm.

c. Invasion of the Ying and Xue systems by pathogenic factor.

Treatment principle: To cool blood, clear heat in the heart, produce body fluid and subdue Yang.

Recipe: Xijiao Dihuang Tang (Decoction of Cornu Rhinoceri Asiatici and Radix Rehmanniae), Zengye Tang (Decoction for Producing Fluid).

Prescription:

3 g of Xijiao (Cornu Rhinoceri Asiatici), or 30 g of buffalo horn

10 g of Shengdi (Radix Rehmanniae)

10 g of Danpi (Cortex Moutan Radicis)

10 g of Danshen (Radix Salviae Miltiorrhizae)

10 g of Xuanshen (Radix Scrophulariae)

10 g of Maidong (Radix Ophiopogonis)

10 g of Longgu (Os Draconis)

10 g of Muli (Concha Ostreae)

Explanation: Xijiao Dihuang Tang clears heat in the Ying system and cools blood. Zengye Tang nourishes and produces body fluid.

Acupuncture treatment: Xijiao, Shengdi, Danpi and Danshen clear heat in the Ying system and cool blood. Xuanshen, Maidong, Longgu and Muli produce body fluid and suppress yang.

A. High fever: Needle Dazhui (Du 14) and Quchi (L.I. 11). If sweating is present, add Fuliu (K. 7). To prick Shaoshang (Lu. 11), Shangyang (L.I. 1) and Shixuan (Extra.) to cause bleeding also lowers body temperature.

B. Convulsion: Needle Renzhong (Du 26), Hegu (L.I. 4), or Houxi (S.I. 3) and Taichong (Liv. 3) as well with moderate stimulation.

C. Respiratory failure: Needle Huiyin (Ren 1) and Suliao (Du 25) with strong stimulation. Needles are retained and manipulated once every 10-20 minutes. Moxibustion is applied to Shanzhong (Ren 17).

Discussion

It is significant to control the syndrome of the Wei stage from developing to the Qi, Ying and Xue stages. The combination of herbal decoction and acupuncture shortens the duration of treatment and reduces after-effects.

The sick child should be helped turn in bed frequently, and the back must be patted now and then. The mouth of the sick child should be kept clean. If retention of urine occurs, acupuncture, massage therapy, or catheterization should be applied.

10. Infantile Paralysis

Infantile paralysis, known as poliomyelitis in Western medicine, is a common infectious disease of children marked by fever, muscular pain, and then paralysis of the limbs. This disease often occurs in summer and autumn, occasionally in spring, more commonly in children between one and five years of age. Thanks to live poliomyelitis vaccination, the incidence of this disease has decreased markedly over the past few years in China.

This disease falls into the category of acute febrile disease, before paralysis occurs at the early stage; and into the category of Wei syndrome, when paralysis occurs.

This disease is caused by invasion of seasonal pestilential factors such as wind, heat, summer heat and damp via the mouth and nose. The Lung and Stomach channels are affected at the early stage. Invasion of the channels and collaterals by pestilential factors leads to weakness of the muscles and motor impairment of joints. Poor circulation of Qi and blood in a prolonged case deprives the tendons, bones and muscles of nourishment, and thereby results in after-effects such as muscular atrophy and deformity of bones and joints.

Differentiation

The entire process of the disease is divided into three syndromes, invasion of the lung and stomach by pathogenic factors, invasion of the channels and collaterals by pathogenic factors, and deficiency of Qi with stagnation of blood. At the early stage of the disease, there is pain in the limbs and trunk, which then disappears, while paralysis emerges. This is different from Bi syndrome which is marked by pain in the four limbs all the time with restricted movements of the joints.

a. Invasion of the lung and stomach by pathogenic factors.

Clinical manifestations: Fever, cough, runny nose, inflamed throat, general malaise, possibly vomiting and loose stool, a red tongue with thin and sticky coating, and a rapid pulse.

Analysis: This syndrome occurs at the early stage when the lung and stomach are diseased at the same time. Invasion of the lung by pathogenic factor impairs its function in descending, and thereby results in fever, cough, runny nose and inflamed throat. Retention of damp-heat in the spleen and stomach impairs their function in ascending and descending with the result of vomiting and loose stool. A red tongue with thin and sticky coating and a rapid pulse are both signs of wind, damp and heat.

b. Invasion of the channels and collaterals by pathogenic factors.

Clinical manifestations: Recurrence of fever, profuse sweating, pain in the limbs and trunk, reluctance to be patted and held, crying, restlessness, a red tongue with thin, sticky and slightly yellow coating, and a weak-floating and rapid pulse.

Analysis: When pathogenic factors are transmitted

inward, heat disappears but damp remains. Damp then turns into heat, and thereby gives rise to retention of damp-heat in the interior. This explains recurrence of fever and profuse sweating. Invasion of the channels and collaterals by damp-heat causes derangement of Qi, which is the cause of pain in the limbs and trunk, reluctance to be patted and held, and restlessness with crying. A red tongue with thin, sticky and slightly yellow coating, and a weak-floating and rapid pulse are signs of damp-heat.

c. Deficiency of Qi with stagnation of blood.

Clinical manifestations: Subsidence of fever, weakness and paralysis of the limbs and trunk, pale complexion, possibly sweating, a pale tongue with thin coating, and a thready and weak pulse.

Analysis: This syndrome manifests as disappearance of pathogenic factors and deficiency of body resistance. Deficiency of Qi with stagnation of blood deprives the tendons and muscles of nourishment, and thereby results in weakness and paralysis of the limbs and trunk. Deficiency of Qi and blood in a prolonged case leads to pale complexion. A pale tongue with thin coating, and a thready and weak pulse are both signs of deficiency of Qi and blood.

Treatment

Chinese herbal medicine:

a. Invasion of the lung and stomach by pathogenic factors.

Treatment principle: To relieve the exterior symptoms, clear heat, eliminate wind and dispel damp.

Recipe: Gegen Huangqin Huanglian Tang (Decoction of Radix Puerariae, Radix Scutellariae and Rhizoma Coptidis).

Prescription:

10 g of Gegen (Radix Puerariae)

10 g of Huangqin (Radix Scutellariae)

2 g of Huanglian (Rhizoma Coptidis)

10 g of Sangye (Folium Mori)

5 g of Qianhu (Radix Peucedani)

5 g of Qianghuo (Rhizoma seu Radix Notopterygii)

10 g of Duhuo (Radix Angelicae Pubescentis)

Explanation: Gegen relieves the exterior symptoms and disperses wind. Huangqin and Huanglian clear heat and relieve toxins, and also dry out damp with bitter and cold nature. Sangye and Qianhu disperse wind-heat. Qianghuo and Duhuo relieve the exterior symptoms and dispel damp.

b. Invasion of the channels and collaterals by pathogenic factors.

Treatment principle: To clear heat, resolve damp, and remove obstruction from channels.

Recipe: Sanmiao Wan (Pill of Three Ingredients with Wonderful Effects).

Prescription:

10 g of Huangbai (Cortex Phellodendri)

10 g of Cangzhu (Rhizoma Atractylodis)

10 g of Niuxi (Radix Achyranthis Bidentatae)

5 g of Fangji (Radix Stephaniae Tetrandrae)

10 g of Qinjiao (Radix Gentiane Macrophyllae)

10 g of Haifengteng (Caulis Piperis Futokadsurae)

10 g of Cansha (Excrementum Bombycis)

Explanation: Huangbai is bitter and cold in nature, and clears heat. Cangzhu, bitter and warm in nature, dries out damp. Niuxi circulates Qi and blood in channels. Fangji, Qinjiao, Haifengteng and Cansha dispel damp and remove obstruction in collaterals.

c. Deficiency of Qi with stagnation of blood.

Treatment principle: To tonify Qi, nourish blood, activate blood circulation and remove obstruction in collaterals.

Recipe: Buyang Huanwu Tang (Decoction for Treating Paralysis).

Prescription:

10 g of Huangqi (Radix Astragali)

10 g of Danggui (Radix Angelicae Sinensis)

3 g of Chuanxiong (Rhizoma Ligustici Chuanxiong)

10 g of Chishao (Radix Paeoniae Rubra)

10 g of Taoren (Semen Persicae)

10 g of Dilong (Lumbricus)

5 g of Honghua (Flos Carthami)

Explanation: This prescription is commonly used in the treatment of Wei syndrome (paralysis), acting to tonify Qi and blood, activate blood circulation and remove obstuction in the channels. Huangqi tonifies Qi. Danggui, Chuanxiong and Chishao nourish blood and activate blood circulation. Taoren, Honghua and Dilong correct blood stasis and remove obstruction in the channels and collaterals.

Acupuncture treatment:

Treatment of paralysis.

A. Upper limbs: Huatuo Jiaji (Extra.), Jianyu (L.I. 15), Jianzhen (S.I. 15), Quchi (L.I. 11), Waiguan (S.J. 5), Hegu (L.I. 4).

B. Lower limbs: Huantiao (G.B. 30), Fengshi (G.B. 31), Zusanli (St. 36), Femur-Futu (St. 32), Yanglingquan (G.B. 34), Yinlingquan (Sp. 9), Kunlun (U.B. 60), Taixi (K. 3), Shenshu (U.B. 23), Yaoyangguan (Du 3). In the case of eversion, needle points at the medial aspect of the leg such as Sanyinjiao (Sp. 6) and Shangqiu (Sp. 5). In the case of inversion, needle points at the lateral aspect of the leg such as Xuanzhong (G.B. 39) and Qiuxu (G.B. 40).

C. Facial nerve: Jiache (St. 6), Dicang (St. 4), Hegu (L.I. 4).

D. Diaphragm: Geshu (U.B. 17), Qimen (Liv. 14), Jiuwei (Ren 15).

E. Abdominal muscle: Zhongwan (Ren 12), Tianshu (St. 25), Qihai (Ren 6).

F. Sphincter vesicae: Shenshu (U.B. 23), Pangguangshu (U.B. 28), Zhongji (Ren 3), Guanyuan (Ren 4), Yinlingquan (Sp. 9).

All the above points are needled with the even method.

Discussion

When the disease develops to paralysis, application of acupuncture is conducive to the recovery, and also reduces the incidence of after-effects. Some sick children with more than one year's duration of disease can still expect improvement with the help of acupuncture.

The syndrome of invasion of the lung and stomach by pathogenic factors presents similar symptoms and signs to the common cold. It is necessary to differentiate them. The common cold usually lasts for about one week, and fever does not occur again once it subsides. If double quotidian fever and pain in the limbs and trunk are present, the possibility of this disease is great.

The sick child at the early stage of the disease should rest in bed absolutely in order to reduce the possibility of paralysis. The sick child should be isolated for one week from both respiratory and digestive aspects, and for 40 days with respect to the digestion.

11. Epidemic Toxic Dysentery

Epidemic toxic dysentery is a severe dysentery marked by abrupt onset of high fever, coma, recurrent convulsion, and visible or invisible dysentery. This disease occurs in summer and autumn in children between two and ten years of age, especially those between two and five years of age. Since the duration of the disease is short, pathological conditions are critical, and mortality is high, it is necessary to establish a correct diagnosis at the early stage of the disease so that treatment will not be delayed.

The pathogenesis of the disease is intake of unclean food, which allows toxic damp and heat to invade the intestinal tract.

Differentiation

When diagnosis of the disease is established, efforts should be made to differentiate tense and flaccid syndromes. The former is due to invasion of the interior of the body by heat toxins disturbing the Liver Channel, while the latter results from weakness of body resistance in contending with the invading pathogenic factors with the result of abrupt collapse of Yang Qi of the body.

a. Tense syndrome due to invasion of the interior of the body by toxins.

Clinical manifestations: High fever, vomiting, restlessness, coma, recurrence of convulsion, dysentery with pus and blood in stool or invisible dysentery in which pus and blood are found in stool through anal finger examination or enema, a red tongue with yellow and coarse coating, and a rolling and rapid pulse.

Analysis: This syndrome is due to invasion of the

stomach and intestines by damp-heat toxins. Upward disturbance of turbid Qi in the stomach leads to vomiting. Downward invasion of toxic heat is the cause of dysentery with pus and blood in the stool or invisible dysentery. When damp-heat toxins turn into fire, high fever and restlessness will occur. Invasion of the pericardium by toxins leads to coma. Disturbance of the Liver Channel by heat produces recurrent convulsion. A red tongue is due to excessive heat. A yellow and coarse coating is due to retention of damp-heat in the interior consuming body fluid. A rolling and rapid pulse is a sign of heat of the excess type.

b. Tense syndrome in the interior with flaccid symptoms on the exterior.

Clinical manifestations: Together with high fever and convulsion, there occur suddenly pale complexion, cold limbs, shortness of breath, indifference, petechiae like decorations on the skin, a pale tongue with yellow coating, and a deep, thready and rapid, or deep, feeble and short pulse.

Explanation: This syndrome is due to weakness of body resistance in contending with invading pathogenic factors, which allows heat toxins to block the interior of the body, while Yang Qi collapses abruptly on the exterior of the body. Feebleness of Yang Qi fails to send Qi and blood to nourish upward, which is the cause of pale complexion. When Yang Qi is unable to warm and nourish muscles and skin, there occur cold limbs or petechiae like decorations on the skin due to stagnation of Qi and blood. Abrupt collapse of Yang Qi also means fading of lung Qi and thereby causes shortness of breath. Deficiency of heart Qi implies impairment of the function of the heart in housing the mind, which causes indifference. Hyperactivity of heat toxins leads to high fever and a yellow tongue coating. Extreme heat produces wind, which is the cause of convulsion. A pale tongue, and a deep, thready and rapid, or deep, feeble and short pulse are signs of prostration.

Treatment

Chinese herbal medicine:

a. Tense syndrome due to invasion of the interior of the body by toxins.

Treatment principle: To clear heat in the intestines, relieve toxins, and promote mental resuscitation.

Recipe: Huanglian Jiedu Tang (Decoction of Rhizoma Coptidis for Relieving Toxins).

Prescription:

3 g of Huanglian (Rhizoma Coptidis)

10 g of Huangqin (Radix Scutellariae)

10 g of Huangbai (Cortex Phellodendri)

10 g of Dahuang (Radix et Rhizoma Rhei), to be decocted later

10 g of Zhishi (Fructus Aurantii Immaturus)

10 g of Gouteng (Ramulus Uncariae cum Uncis)

5 g of Changpu (Rhizoma Acori Graminei)

Explanation: This prescription clears heat in the intestines, reduces fire and relieves toxins. Huangqin, Huanglian and Huangbai reduce fire and relieve toxins. Dahuang and Zhishi clear heat in the intestines and move the bowels. Gouteng and Changpu eliminate wind and promote mental resuscitation.

If vomiting is pronounced, add Yushu Dan (Jade Pivot Pill), to be taken separately, in order to dispel the stale, relieve toxins and check vomiting.

b. Tense syndrome in the interior with flaccid symptoms on the exterior.

Treatment principle: To strengthen body resistance, rescue prostration, subdue Yang and calm wind.

Recipe: Shen Fu Tang (Decoction of Radix Ginseng and Radix Aconiti Praeparata) or Shen Fu Long Mu Jiuni Tang (Decoction of Radix Ginseng, Radix Aconiti Praeparata, Os Draconis and Concha Ostreae for Rescuing the Collapsing State).

Prescription:

10 g of Renshen (Radix Ginseng)

10 g of Shufuzi (Radix Aconiti Praeparata)

10 g of Baishao (Radix Paeoniae Alba)

5 g of Zhigancao (Radix Glycyrrhizae, treated)

20 g of Longgu (Os Draconis)

20 g of Muli (Concha Ostreae)

10 g of Gouteng (Ramulus Uncariae cum Uncis)

20 g of Shijueming (Concha Haliotidis)

Explanation: This prescription recaptures Yang, tonifies Qi and rescues the collapsing state. Renshen and Shufuzi tonify Qi and recapture Yang. Baishao and Gancao protect Yin. Longgu and Muli subdue Yang. Gouteng and Shijueming cool the liver and calm wind.

Tense and flaccid syndromes are treated at the same time. Shen Fu Tang or Shen Fu Long Mu Jiuni Tang is administered first to recapture Yang and rescue the collapsing state. Then Angong Niuhuang Wan (Calculus Bovis Pill for Regaining Mental Clarity) is administered to relieve convulsion and promote mental clarity. When the collapsing state is rescued, Huanglian Jiedu Tang (Decoction of Rhizoma Coptidis for Relieving Toxins) and Baitouweng Tang (Radix Pulsatillae Decoction) are administered for clearing heat in the intestines and checking dysentery.

Acupuncture treatment:

Treatment principle: To clear heat and refresh the brain.

Main points: Renzhong (Du 26) L, Baihui (Du 20) L, Zhongchong (P. 9) L, Neiguan (P. 6) L, Fengchi (G.B. 20) L, Yongquan (K. 1) L, Tianshu (St. 25) L, Shangjuxu (St. 37) L.

Method: When convulsion occurs, needle Renzhong (Du 26) and Baihui (Du 20) first. If these two points are not effective, needle Neiguan (P. 6) and Fengchi (G.B. 20). When coma occurs, needle Renzhong (Du 26) and Zhongchong (P. 9) and the needles are manipulated once every four to five minutes. If there is no response after three to four times of manipulation, needle Neiguan (P. 6), Fengchi (D.B. 20) and Yongquan (K. 1) or apply moxibustion on Qihai (Ren 6) X, Baihui (Du 20) and Shenque (Ren 8) △ 5. If there is pus and blood in the stool, needle Tianshu (St. 25) and Shangjuxu (St. 37). If tenesmus is present, needle Yinlingquan (Sp. 9) 1, Changqiang (Du 1) 1.

Discussion

Since this disease has high mortality in the first two days, early diagnosis and treatment is essential. A combined method in the treatment is conducive to the recovery.

The respiratory tract should be kept free of obstruction. Sufficient water and nourishment should be supplied. See to it that pathological conditions of the sick child are observed closely, such as complexion, respiration, blood pressure and pupils.

12. Summer Fever

Summer fever is a children's disease marked by prolonged fever, thirst with desire to drink large quantities of water, profuse urine and absence of sweating. This disease occurs in summer, in children with weak body constitution between two and five years of age, especially those under three, and is more often seen in southeast and south parts of China.

The internal causative factor of the disease is weakness of body resistance and poor nourishment supply, while the external cause is scorching heat in summer.

When the body resistance is weak, pathogenic summer heat takes the chance to invade the lung and stomach directly. Retention of summer heat in the interior of the body consumes body fluid and thereby causes fever and thirst with desire to drink large quantities of water. Summer heat also consumes Qi and thus impairs the function of the spleen and kidney in transforming and transporting body fluid and dominating water metabolism with the result of discharge of clear and profuse urine. Since fluid of the lung is consumed by summer heat, and the pores are closed, there is not sweating or only little sweating. Both sweat and urine belong to Yin fluid of the body, and they are of the same origin. Thus, absence of sweating leads to profuse urine. Excessive urine consumes Yin fluid, thereby giving rise to thirst with desire to drink large quantities of water. However, deficiency of Qi of the spleen and kidney allows downward movement of body fluid and thus results in profuse urine again. Therefore, body fluid is consumed again and no sweat is produced. Absence of sweating does not allow heat to be dispelled, and persistent fever further consumes body fluid. In this way, fever, absence of sweating, thirst with desire to drink large quantities of water, and profuse urine form a noxious cycle.

Differentiation

The early stage of the disease involves the lung and stomach, while a prolonged illness damages the spleen and kidney.

a. Invasion of the lung and stomach by summer heat.

Clinical manifestations: Persistent fever which rises when atmospheric temperature rises, thirst with desire to drink, a burning sensation of the skin, absence of sweating or only little sweating, profuse urine which is light yellow in colour, restlessness and irritability, dryness of the lips, a red tongue with thin and yellow coating, and a rapid pulse.

Analysis: Invasion of the lung and stomach by summer heat consumes body fluid and produces internal heat, which explains persistent fever, absence of sweating, thirst with desire to drink, and restlessness and irritability. Acted on by increasing high atmospheric temperature, fever goes up accordingly. Summer heat consumes qi, which then fails to transform water, and thus allows water to flow downward to the urinary bladder with the result of profuse and light yellow urine. A red tongue with thin and yellow coating and a rapid pulse are both signs of heat.

b. Excess on the top and deficiency in the bottom.

Clinical manifestations: A prolonged duration of disease, persistent fever, absence of sweating or only little sweating, thirst with desire to drink large quantities of water, clear urine with increased volume and frequency, poor appetite, loose stool, listlessness or restlessness, pale complexion, cold lower limbs, a pale tongue with thin and yellow coating, and a thready, rapid and weak pulse.

Analysis: This is a complicated syndrome of deficiency and excess with prolonged duration, manifesting as invasion of the lung and stomach by summer heat as well as deficiency of Yang of the spleen and kidney. Deficiency of Yang of the spleen and kidney gives rise to pale complexion, listlessness, cold lower limbs, reduced appetite, loose stool, clear urine with increased volume and frequency. A pale tongue with thin and yellow coating, and a thready, rapid and weak pulse are signs of complication between deficiency and excess.

Treatment

Invasion of the lung and stomach is marked by a short duration of the disease with mild pathological conditions, while excess on the top and deficiency in the bottom have a prolonged duration and severe pathological conditions.

Chinese herbal medicine:

a. Invasion of the lung and stomach by summer heat.

Treatment principle: To clear summer heat and tonify Qi.

Recipe: Qingshu Yiqi Tang (Decoction for Clearing Summer Heat and Tonifying Qi).

Prescription:

5 g of Xiyangshen (Western Ginseng)

2 g of Huanglian (Rhizoma Coptidis)

10 g of Maidong (Radix Ophiopogonis)

10 g of Shihu (Herba Dendrobii)

5 g of Zhimu (Rhizoma Anemarrhenae)

5 g of Gancao (Radix Glycyrrhizae)

1/3 of a metre of Hegeng (Ramulus Nelumbinis)

30 g of watermelon peel

Explanation: This prescription clears summer heat, tonifies Qi, nourishes Yin and produces body fluid.

Huanglian, Hegeng and watermelon peel clear heat and relieve toxins. Xiyangshen, which can be replaced by Beishashen (Radix Glehniae), Maidong, Shihu, Zhimu and Gancao tonify Qi and produce body fluid.

b. Excess on the top and deficiency in the bottom.

Treatment principle: To warm the bottom and clear heat on the top.

Recipe: Wenxia Qingshang Tang (Decoction for Warming the Bottom and Clearing Heat on the Top).

Prescription:

5 g of Shufuzi (Radix Aconiti Praeparata)

1 g of Huanglian (Rhizoma Coptidis)

20 g of Shigao (Gypsum Fibrosum)

10 g of Gejie (Gecko)

10 g of Longchi (Dens Draconis)

10 g of Cishi (Magnetitum)

10 g of Buguzhi (Fructus Psoraleae)

10 g of Tusizi (Semen Cuscutae)

10 g of Fupenzi (Fructus Rubi)

10 g of Sangpiaoxiao (Ootheca Mantidis)

10 g of Suoquan Wan (Pill for Reducing Urine), to be decocted, wrapped

Explanation: This prescription clears heat, protects Yin, warms the kidney and subdues Yang. Shufuzi warms Yang in the bottom. Huanglian clears heat on the top. Shigao and Gejie clear heat, produce body fluid and relieve thirst. Longchi and Cishi subdue Yang. Buguzhi, Tusizi, Fupenzi, Sangpiaoxiao and Suoquan Wan warm the kidney, control urine and protect Yin fluid.

Acupuncture treatment:

Treatment principle: To clear heat in general and summer heat in particular.

Points: Dazhui (Du 14) L, Quchi (L.I. 11) L, Sanyinjiao

(Sp. 6) 1, Shenshu (U.B. 23) 1, Qihai (Ren 6) 1.

Discussion

Summer fever is due to weak body resistance of children complicated with invasion by pathogenic summer heat, and is different from infectious febrile diseases in summer. Although high fever is present in summer fever, the invading summer heat does not turn into fire, and there is no invasion of the Ying (nutrient) and Xue (blood) systems.

To avoid summer heat is the best method of prevention and treatment of summer fever. If the sick child is taken away from summer heat stricken areas, high fever will be lowered immediately.

Chapter III
Neonatal Diseases

1. Jaundice of Newborns

Jaundice of newborns is marked by yellowness of the skin, the whites of the eyes and urine. Since most newborns develop jaundice two to four days after birth, ancient scholars thought this disease was related to the mother. Jaundice in older children and adults is pathological, while that in newborns is mostly physiological. Only a small proportion of the cases of newborns' jaundice is pathological. Physiological jaundice does not need treatment and will subside spontaneously. Pathological jaundice should be treated actively.

This disease is due to exposure of the pregnant woman to pathogenic damp-heat which transmits to the fetus, or to direct invasion of the newborn by pathogenic damp-heat. Congenital deficiency of spleen Yang of the fetus is also a causative factor, because this allows transmission of damp from the mother to the fetus. Direct invasion of the newborn by pathogenic cold-damp leads to jaundice as well.

Differentiation

Damp-heat and cold-damp are differentiated according to the duration of the disease and the colour of jaundice. Jaundice due to damp-heat is of short duration, and is bright-yellow in colour, while jaundice due to cold-damp is of long duration, and is dark-yellow in colour.

a. Excess of damp-heat.

Clinical manifestations: Bright yellow skin, face and sclera, scanty and deep-yellow urine, constipation, abdominal distension and fullness, possibly fever, a red tongue with yellow and sticky coating, and a purple capillary vessel of the finger.

Explanation: This syndrome is due to retention of damp-heat in the interior, which impairs the function of the liver and gall bladder in maintaining the free flow of Qi, and thereby spreads the bile on the body surface. This explains the bright-yellow skin like orange peel. Since the body resistance is still strong, the spirit of the sick child is not diminished. The downward movement of damp-heat into the urinary bladder leads to deep-yellow urine like strong tea. Retention of damp-heat in the intestines impairs the function of transmission, and thereby results in dry stool or constipation, and distending pain in the abdomen. A red tongue with yellow and sticky coating, and a purple capillary vessel, are both signs of retention of damp-heat in the interior. This syndrome is also referred to as Yang jaundice.

b. Blockage by cold-damp.

Clinical manifestations: Dark-yellow skin, face and sclera, diminished spirit, anorexia or nausea and vomiting, loose and grey-white stool, cold limbs, a pale tongue with white and sticky coating, and a pale capillary vessel of the finger.

Explanation: This syndrome is due to blockage of the middle Jiao by cold-damp, which results in deficiency of spleen Yang and dysfunction of the spleen in transportation and transformation. As a result, there occurs dark-yellow skin, face and sclera, loose and grey-white stool, cold limbs and vomiting. Diminished spirit is due to weakness of body resistance. A pale tongue with white and sticky coating, and a pale capillary vessel are both signs of deficiency of spleen Qi failing to resolve pathogenic damp. This syndrome is also referred to as Yin jaundice.

Treatment

Chinese herbal medicine.

a. Excess of damp-heat.

Treatment principle: To clear heat and dispel damp.

Recipe: Yinchenhao Tang (Decoction of Herba Artemisiae Scopariae).

Prescription:

10 g of Yinchen (Herba Artemisiae Scopariae)

5 g of Chaoshanzhi (Fructus Gardeniae, fried)

5 g of Dahuang (Radix et Rhizoma Rhei), to be decocted later.

Explanation: Yinchenhao Tang proves effective in the treatment of Yang jaundice. Yinchen is a principal herb for clearing heat and dispelling damp. Shanzhi clears damp-heat in Sanjiao. Dahuang relieves constipation by dispelling heat and relieving toxins. This prescription stresses clearing heat. Once damp-heat is dispelled, jaundice is relieved.

b. Blockage by cold-damp.

Treatment principle: To warm the middle Jiao and resolve damp.

Recipe: Yinchen Lizhong Tang (Decoction of Herba Artemisiae Scopariae for Regulating the Middle Jiao).

Prescription:

10 g of Yinchen (Herba Artemisiae Scopariae)

3 g of Ganjiang (Rhizoma Zingiberis)

10 g of Chaodangshen (Radix Codonopsis Pilosulae, fried)

10 g of Chaobaizhu (Rhizoma Atractylodis Macrocephalae, fried)

10 g of Fuling (Poria)

Explanation: Yinchen clears heat, dispels damp and relieves jaundice. The other herbs warm and invigorate spleen Yang in order to dispel damp.

Discussion

Since Qi and Yin of newborns are weak and Zang-Fu organs are delicate, it is not advisable to prescribe excessive amounts of bitter and cold herbs. Herbs with mild action are used to invigorate the spleen. In the treatment of liver disorders, the spleen and stomach should be considered. This is very important for babies.

Jaundice or hepatitis of a pregnant woman should be treated as early as possible in order to prevent infection. The umbilicus, buttocks and skin of the newborn should be kept clean and free of damage.

2. Erysipelas

Erysipelas is marked by inflamed skin which has a clear border and moves like clouds in the sky. This disease occurs in both adults and children, especially newborns who have a high incidence of the disease with severe pathological conditions.

Erysipelas of newborns is caused by factors before and after birth. Factors before birth refer to diseases of expectant mothers due to exposure to external toxins, while those after birth refer to improper nursing and skin injury which allows invasion by external toxins. Skin injury includes dampness and ulcers of the umbilicus, eczema of the buttocks, and insect bites.

Differentiation

The following two syndromes of erysipelas are both of the excess type. If the disease has a fixed location and is free of systemic symptoms and signs, the pathological condition is mild.

a. Wind-heat toxins.

Clinical manifestations: Redness, swelling and burning pain of the local skin, the eruption moving like clouds in the sky, fever, restlessness, crying, dryness of the mouth and lips, a red tongue with thin and yellow coating, a purple capillary vessel spreading to wind gate or Qi gate.

Analysis: This syndrome is due to invasion of the channels and collaterals by wind-heat toxins, which stir Qi and blood and manifests on the skin surface. This is also the reason for redness, swelling and burning pain of the local skin. Retention of heat toxins in the interior leads to fever, restlessness, and dryness of the mouth and lips. Since wind occurs in gusts and is characterized by rapid change, the invading pathogenic factor circulates with Qi and blood in the channels. Therefore, erysipelas has no fixed location.

b. Invasion of the Ying (nutrient) system by toxins.

Clinical manifestations: Persistent high fever, and redness, pain and burning sensation of the local skin. In severe cases, hemorrhagic spots or blisters or even erosions are seen on the affected skin, and mental cloudiness and convulsion are possible at the same time. The tongue is deep-red with yellow and coarse coating. A purple and dim capillary vessel spreads to vital gate of the finger.

Analysis: Excessive toxins in the interior of the body gives rise to high fever. Invasion of the Ying (nutrient) system by heat toxins creates a burning sensation of the skin accompanied by hemorrhagic spots and skin erosions. Invasion of the pericardium by toxins leads to mental cloudiness. Stirring of liver wind causes convulsion. A deep-red tongue with yellow and coarse coating, and a purple and dim capillary vessel are both signs of excessive toxins.

Treatment

Oral administration of herbal decoction is combined with external application of drugs in the treatment.

Chinese herbal medicine.

a. Wind-heat toxins.

Treatment principle: To eliminate wind, clear heat, reduce fire and relieve toxins.

Recipe: Huanglian Jiedu Tang (Decoction of Rhizoma Coptidis for Relieving Toxins)

Prescription:

10 g of Huangqin (Radix Scutellariae)

2 g of Huanglian (Rhizoma Coptidis)

5 g of Huangbai (Cortex Phellodendri)

5 g of Chaoshanzhi (Fructus Gardeniae, fried)

10 g of Niubangzi (Fructus Arctii)

5 g of Fangfeng (Radix Ledebouriellae)

Explanation: This prescription has a strong effect in reducing fire and relieving toxins. Huangqin, Huanglian, Huangbai and Shanzhi are bitter and cold in nature, and thus reduce fire, clear heat and relieve toxins. Niubangzi and Fangfeng eliminate wind and disperse pathogenic factors.

b. Invasion of the Ying (nutrient) system by toxins.

Treatment principle: To cool blood, relieve toxins, promote mental resuscitation and calm wind.

Recipe: Qingwen Baidu Yin (Decoction for Clearing Evil Heat and Relieving Toxins).

Prescription:

1 g of Xijiao (Cornu Rhinoceri Asiatici)

10 g of Shengdi (Radix Rehmanniae)

10 g of Danpi (Cortex Moutan Radicis)

10 g of Chishao (Radix Paeoniae Rubra)

20 g of Shigao (Gypsum Fibrosum)

10 g of Huangqin (Radix Scutellariae)

5 g of Chaoshanzhi (Fructus Gardeniae, fried)

10 g of Gouteng (Ramulus Uncariae cum Uncis)

5 g of Changpu (Rhizoma Aconi Graminei)

Explanation: This prescription reduces fire, relieves toxins, cools blood and rescues Yin. Xijiao, Shengdi, Danpi and Chishao cool blood and relieve toxins. Shigao, Huanglian, Huangqin and Shanzhi reduce fire and relieve toxins. Gouteng and Changpu calm wind and promote mental resuscitation.

External application of drugs: A proper amount of Ruyi Jinhuang San (Golden Yellow Powder for Good Luck) is mixed with decocted broth of Daqingye (Folium Isatidis), and applied externally on the diseased areas with the effect of clearing heat, dispelling toxins, relieving swelling and pain. Therefore, therapeutic results are enhanced. This method is adopted in the treatment of both syndromes of erysipelas.

Discussion

Erysipelas is an acute infectious skin disease characterized by abrupt onset of the disease, rapid changes of pathological conditions and accompaniment of complications. If it is not properly treated, serious consequences will result. Therefore, this disease should not be regarded as a simple skin disease only.

The sick baby should be well looked after. The skin, especially, the umbilicus and buttocks should be kept clean and dry, and free of injury as well. If eczema or skin injury occurs, proper treatment should be given immediately to prevent infection.

3. Tetanus Neonatorum

Tetanus neonatorum is clinically marked by lockjaw, wry smile, convulsion of the four limbs or opisthotonos. This disease usually occurs four to seven days, occasionally a few weeks, after birth. The earlier the disease occurs, the more dangerous it will be. As a disease with high mortality, its prognosis is poor.

Ancient medical scholars thought that tetanus neonatorum is due to invasion of the umbilical cord of the newborn by wind toxins if the cord is not cut long enough nor tied tightly, or to invasion by toxins if the cord is cut with an unclean iron instrument, or is secondary to umbilical ulcers resulting from invasion of the cord by water and damp when the newborn is bathing.

Differentiation

Clinical manifestations: Cyanosis of lips, lockjaw, gurgling with sputum, inability to suck milk, and inability to utter a cry which makes the mouth, eyes and face drawn, producing wry smile; neck rigidity, convulsion of the four limbs, opisthotonos, protrusion of the umbilicus, tightness of the abdomen and a blue capillary vessel of the finger.

Analysis: This syndrome is due to invasion of the umbilicus by wind toxins, which then spread into the channels and collaterals, blocking the defensive and nutrient Qi, causing derangement of Qi and blood, depriving the tendons of nourishment, and subsequently, stirring liver wind. That is why a series of signs relating to wind are presented. The critical sign of suffocation is due to blockage of air passage by phlegm resulting from stagnation of Qi and blood, and liver wind.

Treatment

The pathological conditions of tetanus neonatorum are critical, and the mortality is high. Treatment should be given as early as possible. It is even more important to control convulsion.

Chinese herbal medicine:

Treatment principle: To remove obstruction in the channels and collaterals, calm wind, and relieve convulsion. External application of drugs is used in combination.

Recipe: Cuofeng San (Powder for Scooping Up Wind).

Prescription: Cuofeng San is mixed with Zhulishui (Bamboo Juice obtained by heating) to be taken three to four times a day, two to three grams each time.

Explanation: This prescription has a strong effect in calming wind and relieving convulsion. It also removes obstruction in the channels and collaterals with its aromatic nature. In this prescription, Shexiang (Moschus) circulates channels and collaterals, and relieves lockjaw. Wugong (Scolopendra), Quanxie (Scorpio), Jiangcan (Bombyx Batryticatus) and Gouteng (Ramulus Uncariae cum Uncis) calm wind and relieve convulsion. Zhusha (Cinnabaris) calms the mind. Since decoction lowers the therapeutic results, it is advisable to take this prescription in the form of powder. Zhulishui is effective in the treatment of phlegm, which is manifested in gurgling with sputum in the throat, and is accumulated in the channels and collaterals of the four limbs.

External application of drugs: Qifeng Suokou Fang (Recipe for Tetanus Neonatorum) is applied. This recipe includes 1 Wugong (Scolopendra), 5 Xieshao (Scorpion Tail), 7 Jiangcan (Bombyx Batryticatus), and 1.5 g of Qumai (Herba Dianthi), all of which are ground into powder. Blow 0.3 g of this powder into the nose each time. If this method creates an excessive reaction and the sick baby cries, administer orally 0.6 g of this powder mixed with broth obtained by cooking 1 g of Bohe (Herba Menthae) instead.

Acupuncture treatment:

Treatment principle:

To calm wind and relieve convulsion.

Points: Baihui (Du 20) L, Renzhong (Du 26) L, Shousanli (L.I. 10) L, Hegu (L.I. 4) 1, Yanglingquan (G.B. 24) 1, Taichong (Liv. 3) through to Yongquan (K.1) L.

Moxibustion with garlic.

Pound 30 g of garlic, which is then made into a cake and placed over the umbilicus. Five to six moxa cones are ignited continuously on the cake. Then place a coin-sized moxa wool cake directly on the umbilicus, and fix it with plaster.

Discussion

Early treatment is essential. If the baby is found sucking milk with loose mouth four to seven days after birth, tetanus is possible. An effective measure should be taken immediately to control convulsion.

The sick baby is hypersensitive to outside stimulation.

Vibration, strong light or loud voice may all induce convulsion. Therefore, the sick baby must be isolated in a quiet room with dim light, preferably, in a warm crib. Herbal decoction should be administered bit by bit at short intervals. If convulsion occurs, both milk intake and herbal administration should be discontinued. Sputum should be removed from the trachea in order to prevent suffocation if convulsion is frequent.

4. Disorders of the Umbilical Region

Disorders of the umbilical region include dampness, ulcer, hemorrhage and protrusion of the umbilicus caused by incorrect ligation of umbilical cord, lack of proper nursing, or excessive crying of the baby.

Differentiation

a. Dampness of the umbilicus.

Clinical manifestations: Fluid oozes from the umbilicus after the cord falls off. As a result, the umbilical region is wet, and sometimes slightly inflamed and swollen.

Analysis: This syndrome is due to invasion of the umbilical region by water and damp or to accumulation of urine in the umbilical region. Retention of turbid damp leads to fluid oozing from the umbilicus. If damp turns into heat, inflammation and swelling will occur in the umbilical region.

b. Ulcer of the umbilicus.

Clinical manifestations: Redness, swelling, burning pain, and oozing of pus in the umbilical region. In severe cases, erosion of the umbilicus is accompanied by high fever, restlessness, red lips and dryness of the mouth.

Analysis: This syndrome is due to invasion of the umbilical region by toxins. Accumulation of toxins in the umbilical region leads to redness, swelling, burning pain and oozing of pus there. The invading toxins in the interior of the body turn into heat and fire, and thereby result in high fever, restlessness, redness of lips, and dryness of the mouth.

c. *Hemorrhage of the umbilicus.*

Clinical manifestations: Persistent oozing of blood from the umbilicus; fever, flushed face and burnt lips, dryness of mouth, a red and dry tongue, spitting of blood, bloody stool, purpura; or pale complexion, listlessness, cold limbs, pale lips, and a pale tongue.

Explanation: This syndrome is due to loose ligation of the umbilical cord. If the cord is not tied up again, bleeding will be persistent. Hyperactivity of fire or excess of heat in the interior of the newborn drives blood and produces blood extravasation. The result is oozing of blood from the wound of the umbilical cord accompanied by fever, flushed face, burnt lips, dryness of mouth, and a red tongue. If the newborn has weak body constitution and deficiency of Qi, Qi fails to control blood; and thereby gives rise to oozing of blood from the umbilical cord, accompanied by pale complexion, listlessness, cold limbs, pale lips, and a pale tongue.

d. *Protrusion of the umbilicus.*

Clinical manifestations: Shiny round swelling of the umbilicus, which is as big as a walnut in severe cases, and which will retract on pressure but will protrude again when the baby cries.

Analysis: This syndrome is due to thin and loose muscles of the abdominal wall of the newborn, or to congenital underdevelopment of the newborn, which causes incomplete closure of the umbilical hole. Excessive crying of the newborn allows the panniculus of the small intestines to go into the umbilicus, thus leading to shiny swelling there.

Treatment

***Chinese herbal medicine*:**

a. Dampness of the umbilicus.

Treatment principle: To dry dampness.

Recipe: Shenqi San (Powder for Arresting Oozing of Fluid from the Umbilicus).

Explanation: Longgu (Os Draconis) and Kufan (Alumen, calcined) dry dampness. Shexiang (Moschus), which can be replaced by Bingpian (Borneolum), dispels the stale and regrows muscles. If there is local inflammation, apply Ruyi Jinhuang San (Golden Yellow Powder for Good Luck) externally on the diseased area to clear heat and dispel damp.

b. Ulcer of the umbilicus.

Treatment principle: To clear heat and relieve toxins.

Recipe: Wuwei Xiaodu Yin (Decoction of Five Ingredients for Relieving Toxins).

Prescription:

10 g of Zihuadiding (Herba Violae)

10 g Tiankui (Herba Semiaquilegiae)

10 g of Yinhua (Flos Lonicerae)

10 g of Juhua (Flos Chrysanthemi)

10 g of Pugongying (Herba Taraxaci)

Explanation: All these herbs clear heat, dispel toxins and relieve swelling.

External application of drugs: Wash the diseased area with broth obtained by cooking Fangfeng (Radix Ledebouriellae), Juhua and Yinhua. Then dry the area and apply Ruyi Jinhuang San there.

c. Hemorrhage of the umbilicus.

(1) Loose ligation.

The umbilical cord should be tied up again. Longgu San (Os Draconis Powder) is applied externally to the diseased area.

(2) Excessive heat in the interior.

Treatment principle: To clear heat and cool blood.

Recipe: Qiangen San (Radix Rubiae Powder)

Prescription:

2 g of Huanglian (Rhizoma Coptidis)

10 g of Huangqin (Radix Scutellariae)

5 g of Shanzhi (Fructus Gardeniae)

10 g of Shengdi (Radix Rehmanniae)

5 g of Qiancao (Radix Rubiae)

10 g of Diyu (Radix Sanguisorbae)

Explanation: Huanglian, Huangqin and Shanzhi reduce fire and relieve toxins. Shengdi, Qiancao and Diyu cool blood and check bleeding.

External application of drugs: Ruyi Jinhuang San is applied to the diseased area.

(3) Qi failing to control blood.

Treatment principle: To tonify Qi and control blood.

Recipe: Guipi Tang (Decoction for Restoring the Spleen).

Prescription:

10 g of Dangshen (Radix Codonopsis Pilosulae)

10 g of Huangqi (Radix Astragali)

10 g of Baizhu (Rhizoma Atractylodis Macrocephalae)

5 g of Gancao (Radix Glycyrrhizae)

10 g of Danggui (Radix Angelicae Sinensis)

10 g of Xueyutan (Crinis Carbonisatus)

10 g of Cebaiye (Cacumen Biotae)

Explanation: Dangshen, Huangqi, Baizhu and Gancao tonify Qi and invigorate the spleen; Danggui nourishes blood; Xueyutan and Cebaiye check bleeding.

External application of drugs: Longgu San (Powder of Os Draconis) is applied to the diseased area.

d. Protrusion of the umbilicus.

Oral administration of medicine is unnecessary, external treatment being usually given. Push the protrusion inward, fix it with a hard object like coin, which is wrapped in cotton and gauze, and then have the umbilical region tightly bandaged. With all this done, try to make the newborn cry as little as possible.

If a baby of more than two years old suffers from an umbilical protrusion more than two centimetres in diameter, and does not respond to the above treatment, surgical operation should be performed.

Discussion

Prevention is more important than treatment in dealing with umbilical disorders of the newborn. Proper nursing should be given.

5. Sclerema Neonatorum

Sclerema neonatorum is marked by sclerosis and edema of subcutaneous fat, and is likely to occur in cold seasons, in premature infants or infants with other disorders seven to ten days after birth.

The internal cause of this disease is deficiency of congenital Qi, while the external cause is exposure to cold due to improper nursing. Direct invasion of Zang-Fu organs by external pathogenic cold damages Yang of the spleen and stomach, and thereby does not allow

Yang Qi to warm the muscles and skin with the result of sclerema.

Differentiation

a. Deficiency of Yang Qi.

Clinical manifestations: The body as cold as ice, lying with little movement, drowsiness, feeble breathing, weak cry, difficulty in sucking milk, muscles and skin hard and stiff, sclerema over extensive areas, pale complexion, tongue and lips, and an indistinct reddish capillary vessel of the finger.

Explanation: This syndrome is due to feebleness of kidney Yang with excessive Yin cold in the interior of the body. This explains the body as cold as ice, lying with little movement, drowsiness, feeble breathing, weak cry, and difficulty in sucking milk. Cold, marked by contraction and stagnation, makes the muscles and skin hard and stiff. Pale complexion, tongue and lips, and a reddish capillary vessel are all signs of deficiency of Yang Qi.

b. Stagnation of blood due to invasion by cold.

Clinical manifestations: Cold limbs and body; sclerema which does not allow the skin to be pinched up and which begins in the leg and thigh, then spreads to the buttocks, or even to upper limbs and cheek; the affected skin dark-purple in colour, or red and swollen; sallow complexion, dark-red lips and tongue, and an indistinct deep and dark capillary vessel of the finger.

Analysis: Invasion of the body by external pathogenic cold causes the retardation of Qi and blood circulation, so that Qi and blood are not able to warm and nourish the muscles, skin and limbs. As a result, there occurs cold limbs and body, and sclerema which makes the skin unable to be pinched up. Deficiency of Yang of the spleen and kidney with excessive cold-damp in the interior of the body allows sclerema to begin in the leg and thigh, and then spread upward. Stagnation of blood due to cold produces dark-purple or red and swollen skin. Sallow complexion, dark-red lips and tongue, and an indistinct, deep and dark capillary vessel are all signs of stagnation of blood due to invasion of cold.

Treatment

The method of treatment is to tonify Qi, warm Yang, circulate blood and remove obstruction from the vessels. Other measures should be taken as well to restore normal body temperature and conserve warmth.

Chinese herbal medicine:

a. Deficiency of Yang Qi.

Treatment principle: To tonify Qi and warm Yang.

Recipe: Shen Fu Tang (Decoction of Radix Ginseng and Radix Aconiti Praeparata).

Prescription:

10 g of Renshen (Radix Ginseng)

10 g of Shufuzi (Radix Aconiti Praeparata)

5 g of Guizhi (Ramulus Cinnamomi)

10 g of Huangqi (Radix Astragali)

10 g of Danggui (Radix Angelicae Sinensis)

Explanation: Renshen tonifies congenital Qi greatly. Shufuzi warms Yang and disperses cold. Guizhi warms and circulates Yang Qi. Huangqi and Danggui tonify Qi and activate blood circulation.

b. Stagnation of blood due to invasion by cold.

Treatment principle: To warm the channels and remove obstruction from vessels.

Recipe: Danggui Sini Tang (Radix Angelicae Sinensis Decoction for Treating Vital Prostration with Cold Limbs).

Prescription:

10 g of Danggui (Radix Angelicae Sinensis)
10 g of Chishao (Radix Paeoniae Rubra)
5 g of Guizhi (Ramulus Cinnamomi)
3 g of Xixin (Herba Asari)
5 g of Gancao (Radix Glycyrrhizae)
10 g of Dangshen (Radix Codonopsis Pilosulae)
10 g of Huangqi (Radix Astragali)
5 g of Mutong (Caulis Akebiae)
6 pieces of Dazao (Fructus Ziziphi Jujubae)

Explanation: This prescription warms the channels, disperses cold, nourishes blood, removes obstruction from the vessels, tonifies Qi and assists Yang. Danggui and Chishao nourish blood and activate blood circulation. Guizhi and Xixin warm the channels and disperse cold. Dazao and Gancao tonify the spleen. Mutong removes obstruction from the vessels. Dangshen and Huangqi tonify Qi and assist Yang.

In the treatment of both types, injection of Chuanxiong (Rhizoma Ligustici Chuanxiong) and Honghua (Flos Carthami) fluid, compound Danshen (Radix Salviae Miltiorrhizae) fluid, or Renshen (Radix Ginseng) fluid activates blood circulation, corrects blood stasis, tonifies Qi and warms Yang.

Acupuncture treatment:

If sclerema is relieved slowly, apply moxibustion in stick form to local area.

Other therapies:

To conserve warmth and restore normal body temperature is an important measure in the treatment of sclerema neonatorum. The body temperature should be restored slowly, because abrupt elevation of body temperature may cause bleeding of the lung. The actual methods are as follows:

A. Wrap the sick baby in a warm blanket or cotton quilt, then place the baby in a room with temperature between 21°C and 25°C. The body temperature is measured once every 1-2 hours until it rises to 35°C. Then remove the blanket or cotton quilt.

B. If warm incubator is available, place the sick baby into it with the temperature of 26°C, which is raised 1°C per hour until it reaches 30-32°C, not exceeding 34°C. The relative humidity of the warm incubator is kept at 55 percent.

C. The normal body temperature should be restored within 24 hours.

Discussion

Both oral administration of herbal medicine and the method to restore the normal body temperature are important in the treatment. Careful nursing should be given. Attention should be paid to disinfectant isolation of the sick baby in order to prevent cross infection. For the sick baby with difficulty in sucking milk, drop feeding or adopt nasal feeding.

Appendix

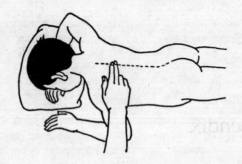

Diagram 1

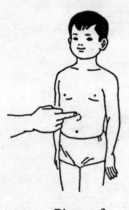

Diagram 3

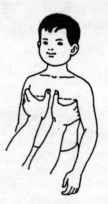

Diagram 2

Chinese Massage Therapy for Children

Chinese massage therapy for children is indicated in certain diseases of children under five years of age. The younger the children are, the more satisfactory the therapeutic results will be. The force used in the treatment of children should be gentle and soft, and the speed of movement is fast. In addition to common points for both adults and children, there are specific massage points for children only.

1. Commonly used techniques for children.

A. Push method.

This technique applies the flat or the side of the thumb, or the flat of the index and middle fingers to slide on certain points in a straight line. (Diag. 1) This technique also uses the flat of both thumbs to slide on the same point in opposite directions. (Diag. 2)

B. Rub method with a circular motion.

Firmly fix the tip of the index finger, the middle finger, or the thumb, or the palm heel on the point and then bring the skin and muscles there into a circular motion. (Diag. 3) The finger tip is employed on a small area, while the palm heel is used on a big area.

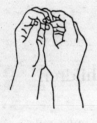

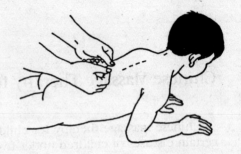

Diagram 4

C. Spinal pinch method.

There are two ways. One of them is described in "Other Therapies" of Chapter III. The other one requires loose fists made with the middle, ring and small fingers of both hands, the index fingers slightly flexed and the thumbs extended in the direction of the distal segment of the index fingers respectively. Then pinch up the skin and muscles over the spinal column with the thumb and index finger. As the two hands alternate in pinching the skin and muscles, the ridge thus formed moves upward from the coccygeal vertebra to Dazhui (Du. 14), which is below the seventh cervical vertebra. (Diag. 4)

D. Spinal push method.

Slide on the spinal column with the flat of the index and middle fingers from Dazhui (Du 14) down to the lumbar vertebrae. (Diag. 5.)

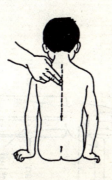

Diagram 5

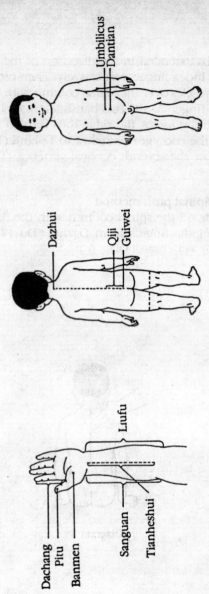

Diagram 6

2. Commonly used points.

Diag. 6 and the following table show the commonly used points for children:

Dachang Pitu Banmen Sanguan Tianheshui Liufu Dazhui Qiji Guiwei Umbilicus Dantian

Diag. 6

Point	Location	Indication	Technique
Pitu	Distal segment of the thumb on palmar side.	Diarrhea, vomiting.	Push 200-500 times.
Da-chang	Radial side of the index finger from tip to web margin.	Retention of food, diarrhea.	Push 100-300 times.
Ban-men	The thenar eminence.	Stuffiness in the chest, vomiting, abdominal fullness due to retention of food, anorexia.	Push or rub with a circular motion 50-200 times.
San-guan	Radial side of the forearm from wrist to elbow.	Aversion to cold, absence of sweating, under-nourishment.	Push 200-500 times from wrist to elbow.
Liufu	Ulnar side of the forearm from wrist to elbow.	Fever and profuse sweating. It is not used for deficiency syndromes.	Push 100-500 times from elbow to wrist.

Tian-heshui	Middle line of medial aspect of forearm from wrist to elbow.	Feverish sensation of body, restlessness, fever due to invasion by external pathogens.	Push 100-500 times from wrist to elbow.
Qiji	A line from 4th lumbar vertebra to coccygeal vertebra.	Diarrhea, dysentery, abdominal distension due to retention of food, constipation due to heat in the intestines.	Push 200-500 times either downward or upward.
Guiwei	Coccygeal vertebra.	Diarrhea, prolapse of anus, constipation.	Rub with a circular motion 300-600 times.
Dantian	2 *cun* below umbilicus.	Pain in lower abdomen, nocturnal enuresis, prolapse of anus, scanty and deep-yellow urine.	Rub with a circular motion for 3-5 minutes.

3. Treatment of commonly seen diseases.

A. Diarrhea: Chinese massage therapy is effective in the treatment of diarrhea. It also renders definite therapeutic results in the treatment of bacillary dysentery, acute and chronic enteritis. Push Pitu 500 times, push Dachang 200 times, rub the abdomen for 5 minutes, rub the umbilicus with a circular motion for 3 minutes, push

Qiji 300 times and rub Guiwei 500 times with a circular motion ; rub Banmen 50 times as well, with a circular motion, for vomiting milk.

B. Gan syndrome (malnutrition): Push Pitu 500 times, push Dachang 200 times, push Sanguan 400 times, rub the abdomen for 5 minutes, and pinch the spine 5 times.

C. Fever due to invasion by external pathogens: Push Tianheshui 300 times, push Liufu 300 times, push the spine 500 times, grasp Fengchi (G.B. 20) and Jianjing (G.B. 21) several times. If fever is not accompanied by sweating, push Sanguan 400 times as well.

D. Prolapse of the anus: Rub Dantian for 5 minutes with a circular motion, rub abdomen for 3 minutes, rub Guiwei 500 times with a circular motion, and push Qiji 300 times.

Index of the Selected Recipes and Patent Medicines

Index of the Selected Recipes and
Patent Medicines

A

Angong Niuhuang Wan (Calculus Bovis Pill for Regaining Mental Clarity)
  Niuhuang (Calculus Bovis)
  Yujin (Radix Curcumae)
  Xijiao (Cornu Rhinoceri)
  Huanglian (Rhizoma Coptidis)
  Zhusha (Cinnabaris)
  Bingpian (Borneolum)
  Zhenzhu (Margarita)
  Shanzhi (Fructus Gardeniae)
  Xionghuang (Realgar)
  Huangqin (Radix Scutellariae)
  Shexiang (Moschus)

B

Baihu Tang (White Tiger Decoction)
  Shigao (Gypsum Fibrosum)
  Zhimu (Rhizoma Anemarrhenae)
  Gancao (Radix Glycyrrhizae)
  Gengmi (Rice)
Baitouweng Tang (Radix Pulsatillae Decoction)
  Baitouweng (Radix Pulsatillae)
  Huangbai (Cortex Phellodendri)
  Huanglian (Rhizoma Coptidis)

Qinpi (Cortex Fraxini)
Baohe Wan (Pill for Protecting Harmony)
    Shanzha (Fructus Crataegi)
    Liuque (Massa Fermentata Medicinalis)
    Banxia (Rhizoma Pinelliae)
    Fuling (Poria)
    Chenpi (Pericarpium Citri Reticulatae)
    Lianqiao (Fructus Forsythiae)
    Laifuzi (Semen Raphani)
    Maiya (Fructus Hordei Germinatus)
Bazhen Tang (Decoction of Eight Pearls)
    Danggui (Radix Angelicae Sinensis)
    Chuanxiong (Rhizoma Ligustici Chuanxiong)
    Baishao (Radix Paeoniae Alba)
    Shudi (Radix Rehmanniae Praeparata)
    Renshen (Radix Ginseng)
    Baizhu (Rhizoma Atractylodis Macrocephalae)
    Fuling (Poria)
    Zhigancao (Radix Glycyrrhizae, treated)
Bing Peng San (Powder of Borneolum Syntheticum and
    Borax)
    Bingpian (Borneolum Syntheticum)
    Duanpengsha (Borax, calcined)
Buyang Huanwu Tang (Decoction for Treating Para-
    lysis)
    Huangqi (Radix Astragali)
    Danggui (Radix Angelicae Sinensis)
    Chishao (Radix Paeoniae Rubra)
    Chuanxiong (Rhizoma Ligustici Chuanxiong)
    Dilonggan (Lumbricus, dry)
    Taoren (Semen Persicae)
    Honghua (Flos Carthami)
Buzhong Yiqi Tang (Decoction for Tonifying the Middle

Jiao and Benefiting Qi)
Huangqi (Radix Astragali)
Renshen (Radix Ginseng)
Baizhu (Rhizoma Atractylodis Macrocephalae)
Gancao (Radix Glycyrrhizae)
Danggui (Radix Angelicae Sinensis)
Chenpi (Pericarpium Citri Reticulatae)
Shengma (Rhizoma Cimicifugae)
Chaihu (Radix Bupleuri)
Shengjiang (Rhizoma Zingiberis Recens)
Dazao (Fructus Ziziphi Jujubae)

C

Cuofeng San (Powder for Scooping Up Wind)
Wugong (Scolopendra)
Gouteng (Ramulus Uncariae cum Uncis)
Xiewei (Scorpio Tail)
Zhusha (Cinnabaris)
Shexiang (Moschus)
Jiangcan (Bombyx Batryticatus)
Zhuli (Bamboo Juice obtained with heating)

D

Dadingfeng Zhu (Precious Decoction for Ceasing Wind)
Baishao (Radix Paeoniae Alba)
Ejiao (Colla Corii Asini)
Guiban (Plastrum Testudinis)
Shengdi (Radix Rehmanniae)
Maren (Fructus Cannabis)

Wuweizi (Fructus Schisandrae)
Muli (Concha Ostreae)
Maidong (Radix Ophiopogonis)
Gancao (Radix Glycyrrhizae)
Jizihuang (Egg yolk)
Biejia (Carapax Trionycis)
Danggui Sini Tang (Radix Angelicae Sinensis Decoction
   for Treating Vital Prostration with Cold Limbs)
Guizhi (Ramulus Cinnamomi)
Xixin (Herba Asari)
Baishao (Radix Paeoniae Alba)
Danggui (Radix Angelicae Sinensis)
Zhigancao (Radix Glycyrrhizae, treated)
Mutong (Caulis Akebiae)
Dazao (Fructus Ziziphi Jujubae)
Dingchuan Tang (Decoction for Soothing Asthma)
Mahuang (Herba Ephedrae)
Baiguo (Semen Ginkgo)
Huangqin (Radix Scutellariae)
Banxia (Rhizoma Pinelliae)
Kuandonghua (Flos Farfarae)
Sangbaipi (Cortex Mori Radicis)
Gancao (Radix Glycyrrhizae)
Xingren (Semen Armeniacae Amarum)
Suzi (Fructus Perillae)
Dingtu Wan (Pill for Checking Vomiting)
Dingxiang (Flos Caryophylli)
Xiewei (Scorpio Tail)
Banxia (Rhizoma Pinelliae),
Zaorou (Fructus Ziziphi Jujubae, meat)
Ding Yu Lizhong Tang (Decoction of Flos Caryophylli
   and Fructus Evodiae for Regulating the Middle Jiao)
Dingxiang (Flos Caryophylli)

238

Wuyu (Fructus Evodiae)
Dangshen (Radix Codonopsis Pilosulae)
Baizhu (Rhizoma Atractylodis Macrocephalae)
Ganjiang (Rhizoma Zingiberis)
Zhigancao (Radix Glycyrrhizae, treated)

E

Erchen Tang (Decoction of Two Old Drugs)
Banxia (Rhizoma Pinelliae)
Chenpi (Pericarpium Citri Reticulatae)
Fuling (Poria)
Zhigancao (Radix Glycyrrhizae, treated)

F

Famu Wan (Lumberjack's Pill)
Zhicangzhu (Rhizoma Atractylodis, treated)
Huangjiuque (yellow rice wine)
Duanzaofan (Melanterite, calcined)

G

Ganji San (Powder for Relieving Stagnation)
Wuguchong (Chrysomyiae Megacephalae)
Shenque (Massa Fermentata Medicinalis)
Binglang (Semen Arecae),
Huhuanglian (Rhizoma Picrorhizae)
Maiya (Fructus Hordei Germinatus)
Xiangfu (Rhizoma Cyperi)
Cangzhu (Rhizoma Atractylodis)

Rouguo (Semen Myristicae).

Gegen Huangqin Huanglian Tang (Decoction of Radix Puerariae, Radix Scutellariae and Rhizoma Coptidis)

Gegen (Radix Puerariae)

Huangqin (Radix Scutellariae)

Huanglian (Rhizoma Coptidis)

Gancao (Radix Glycyrrhizae)

Guipi Tang (Decoction for Restoring the Spleen)

Baizhu (Rhizoma Atractylodis Macrocephalae)

Huangqi (Radix Astragali)

Longyanrou (Arillus Longan)

Fushen (Poria cum Radice Pino)

Suanzaoren (Semen Ziziphi Spinosae)

Dangshen (Radix Codonopsis Pilosulae)

Danggui (Radix Angelicae Sinensis)

Muxiang (Radix Aucklandiae)

Yuanzhi (Radix Polygalae)

Zhigancao (Radix Glycyrrhizae, treated)

Shengjiang (Rhizoma Zingiberis Recens)

Dazao (Fructus Ziziphi Jujubae)

Guizhi Tang (Ramulus Cinnamomi Decoction)

Guizhi (Ramulus Cinnamomi)

Chishao (Radix Paeoniae Rubra)

Gancao (Radix Glycyrrhizae)

Shengjiang (Rhizoma Zingiberis Recens)

Dazao (Fructus Ziziphi Jujubae)

Guzhen Tang (Decoction for Consolidating Yang)

Renshen (Radix Ginseng)

Baizhu (Rhizoma Atractylodis Macrocephalae)

Fuling (Poria)

Zhigancao (Radix Glycyrrhizae, treated)

Huangqi (Radix Astragali)

Paofuzi (Radix Aconiti Praeparata)

Rougui (Cortex Cinnamomi)
Shanyao (Rhizoma Dioscoreae)

H

Huagai San (Powder for Lung Disorders)
　　Mahuang (Herba Ephedrae)
　　Xingren (Semen Armeniacae Amarum)
　　Gancao (Radix Glycyrrhizae)
　　Sangbaipi (Cortex Mori Radicis)
　　Suzi (Fructus Perillae)
　　Chifuling (Poria, red)
　　Chenpi (Pericarpium Citri Reticulatae)
Huanglian Jiedu Tang (Decoction of Rhizoma Coptidis
　　for Relieving Toxins)
　　Huanglian (Rhizoma Coptidis)
　　Huangqin (Radix Scutellariae)
　　Huangbai (Cortex Phellodendri)
　　Shanzhi (Fructus Gardeniae)
Huo Lian Tang (Decoction of Herba Agastachis and
　　Rhizoma Coptidis)
　　Huanglian (Rhizoma Coptidis)
　　Houpo (Cortex Magnoliae Officinalis)
　　Huoxiang (Herba Agastachis)
　　Shengjiang (Rhizoma Zingiberis Recens)
　　Dazao (Fructus Ziziphi Jujubae)
Huoxiang Zhengqi San (Powder of Herba Agastachis for
　　Normalizing Qi)
　　Huoxiang (Herba Agastachis)
　　Suye (Folium Perillae)
　　Baizhi (Radix Angelicae Dahuricae)
　　Jiegeng (Radix Platycodi)

Baizhu (Rhizoma Atractylodis Macrocephalae)
Houpo (Cortex Magnoliae Officinalis)
Banxiaque (Leaven of Rhizoma Pinelliae)
Dafupi (Pericarpium Arecae)
Fuling (Poria)
Chenpi (Pericarpium Citri Reticulatae)
Gancao (Radix Glycyrrhizae)
Shengjiang (Rhizoma Zingiberis Recens)
Dazao (Fructus Ziziphi Jujubae)
Hupo Baolong Wan (Pill of Amber for Holding the Dragon)
Hupo (Amber)
Danxing (Arisaema cum Bile)
Zhusha (Cinnabaris)
Chenxiang (Lignum Aquilariae Resinatum)
Fuling (Poria)
Yueshi (Borax)
Zhuhuang (Bamboo Fungus)
Shanyao (Rhizoma Dioscoreae)
Xionghuang (Realgar)
Zhiqiao (Fructus Aurantii)
Shexiang (Moschus)
Gancao (Radix Glycyrrhizae)

J

Jianpi Wan (Pill for Invigorating the Spleen)
Renshen (Radix Ginseng)
Baizhu (Rhizoma Atractylodis Macrocephalae)
Chenpi (Pericarpium Citri Reticulatae)
Maiya (Fructus Hordei Germinatus)
Shanzha (Fructus Crataegi)

Zhishi (Fructus Aurantii Immaturus)
Shenque (Massa Fermentata Medicinalis)
Jing Fang Baidu San (Powder of Herba Schizonepetae
and Radix Ledebouriellae for Relieving Toxins)
Jingjie (Herba Schizonepetae)
Fangfeng (Radix Ledebouriellae)
Qianghuo (Rhizoma seu Radix Notopterygii)
Duhuo (Radix Angelicae Pubescentis)
Chaihu (Radix Bupleuri)
Chuanxiong (Rhizoma Ligustici Chuanxiong)
Zhiqiao (Fructus Aurantii)
Fuling (Poria)
Gancao (Radix Glycyrrhizae)
Jiegeng (Radix Platycodi)
Qianhu (Radix Peucedani)
Renshen (Radix Ginseng)
Shengjiang (Rhizoma Zingiberis Recens)
Bohe (Herba Menthae)
Jingui Shenqi Wan (Pill for Restoring the Function of
the Kidney)
Gandihuang (Radix Rehmanniae, dry)
Shanyao (Rhizoma Dioscoreae)
Shanzhuyu (Fructus Corni)
Zexie (Rhizoma Alismatis)
Fuling (Poria)
Danpi (Cortex Moutan Radicis)
Fuzi (Radix Aconiti Praeparata)
Guizhi (Ramulus Cinnamomi)

L

Liangge San (Powder for Cooling the Diaphragm)

Dahuang (Radix et Rhizoma Rhei)
Mangxiao (Natrii Sulfas)
Gancao (Radix Glycyrrhizae)
Zhizi (Fructus Gardeniae)
Huangqin (Radix Scutellariae)
Bohe (Herba Menthae)
Lianqiao (Fructus Forsythiae)
Zhuye (Herba Lophatheri)
Baimi (Honey)

Liangying Qingqi Tang (Decoction for Cooling the Ying
System and Clearing Heat in the Qi System)
Xijiaojian (Cornu Rhinoceri Asiatici)
Xianshihu (Herba Dendrobii, fresh)
Shengshigao (Gypsum Fibrosum, raw)
Xianshengdi (Radix Rehmanniae, fresh)
Boheye (Folium Menthae)
Shenggancao (Radix Glycyrrhizae, raw)
Huanglian (Rhizoma Coptidis)
Jiaozhizi (Fructus Gardeniae, burnt)
Danpi (Cortex Moutan Radicis)
Chishao (Radix Paeoniae Rubra)
Xuanshen (Radix Scrophulariae)
Lianqiaoqiao (Fructus Forsythiae)
Xianzhuye (Herba Lophatheri, fresh)
Maogen (Rhizoma Imperatae)
Lugen (Rhizoma Phragmitis)

Jinzhi (Powder of Radix Glycyrrhizae, human faeces
treated)

Lingjiao Gouteng Tang (Decoction of Cornu Antelopis
and Ramulus Uncariae cum Uncis)
Lingyangjiao (Cornu Antelopis)
Sangye (Folium Mori)
Chuanbeimu (Bulbus Fritillariae Cirrhosae)

Shengdi (Radix Rehmanniae)
Gouteng (Ramulus Uncariae cum Uncis)
Juhua (Flos Chrysanthemi)
Shengbaishao (Radix Paeoniae Alba, raw)
Shenggancao (Radix Glycyrrhizae, raw)
Zhuru (Caulis Bambusae in Taenis)
Fushen (Poria cum Radice Pino)
Liujunzi Tang (Decoction of Six Noble Ingredients)
Renshen (Radix Ginseng)
Baizhu (Rhizoma Atractylodis Macrocephalae)
Fuling (Poria)
Gancao (Radix Glycyrrhizae)
Chenpi (Pericarpium Citri Reticulatae)
Banxia (Rhizoma Pinelliae)
Liushen Wan (Pill of Six Ingredients with Magical
Effects)
Shexiang (Moschus)
Niuhuang (Calculus Bovis)
Bingpian (Borneolum)
Zhenzhu (Margarita)
Chansu (Venenum Bufonis)
Xionghuang (Realgar)
Liuwei Dihuang Wan (Pill of Radix Rehmanniae in Six
Ingredients)
Shudi (Radix Rehmanniae Praeparata)
Shanyao (Rhizoma Dioscoreae)
Shanyurou (Fructus Corni)
Fuling (Poria)
Zexie (Rhizoma Alismatis)
Danpi (Cortex Moutan Radicis)
Longgu San (Os Draconis Powder)
Longgu (Os Draconis)
Kufan (Alum, calcined)

M

Mahuang Lianqiao Chixiaodou Tang (Decoction of He-
ba Ephedrae, Fructus Forsythiae and Semen Phaseoli)
    Mahuang (Herba Ephedrae)
    Lianqiao (Fructus Forsythiae)
    Chixiaodou (Semen Phaseoli)
    Xingren (Semen Armeniacae Amarum)
    Shengxinbaipi (Cortex Catakpae Radicis, raw)
    Shengjiang (Rhizoma Zingiberis Recens)
    Dazao (Fructus Ziziphi Jujubae)
    Zhigancao (Radix Glycyrrhizae, treated)
Ma Xing Shi Gan Tang (Decoction of Herba Ephedrae,
Semen Armeniacae Amarum, Gypsum Fibrosum
    and Radix Glycyrrhizae)
    Mahuang (Herba Ephedrae)
    Xingren (Semen Armeniacae Amarum)
    Shigao (Gypsum Fibrosum)
    Gancao (Radix Glycyrrhizae)

N

Niuhuang Qingxin Wan (Calculus Bovis Pill for Clearing
    Heat in the Heart)
    Niuhuang (Calculus Bovis)
    Huangqin (Radix Scutellariae)
    Huanglian (Rhizoma Coptidis)
    Shanzhi (Fructus Gardeniae)
    Yujin (Radix Curcumae)
    Zhusha (Cinnabaris)

P

Puji Xiaodu Yin (Decoction for General Relief and Dispelling Toxins)
Huangqin (Radix Scutellariae)
Huanglian (Rhizoma Coptidis)
Lianqiao (Fructus Forsythiae)
Xuanshen (Radix Scrophulariae)
Banlangen (Radix Isatidis)
Mabo (Lasiosphaera seu Calvatia)
Niubangzi (Fructus Arctii)
Jiangcan (Bombyx Batryticatus)
Shengma (Rhizoma Cimicifugae)
Chaihu (Radix Bupleuri)
Chenpi (Pericarpium Citri Reticulatae)
Jiegeng (Radix Platycodi)
Gancao (Radix Glycyrrhizae)
Renshen (Radix Ginseng) or Bohe (Herba Menthae)

Q

Qiangen San (Radix Rubiae Powder)
Qiangen (Radix Rubiae)
Diyu (Radix Sanguisorbae)
Shengdihuang (Radix Rehmanniae, raw)
Danggui (Radix Angelicae Sinensis)
Zhizi (Fructus Gardeniae)
Huangqin (Radix Scutellariae)
Huanglian (Rhizoma Coptidis)
Xijiao (Cornu Rhinoceri Asiatici)
Qingjie Toubiao Tang (Decoction for Clearing Heat, Relieving Toxins and Bringing the Rash Out)

Xiheliu (Cacumen Tamaricis)
Chanyi (Periostracum Cicadae)
Gegeng (Radix Puerariae)
Shengma (Rhizoma Cimicifugae)
Zicaogen (Radix Arnebiae seu Lithospermi)
Sangye (Folium Mori)
Juhua (Flos Chrysenthemi)
Gancao (Radix Glycyrrhizae)
Niubangzi (Fructus Arctii)
Yinhua (Flos Lonicerae)
Lianqiao (Fructus Forsythiae)
Qingre Xiepi San (Powder for Clearing Heat in the Spleen)
Shanzhi (Fructus Gardeniae)
Shengshigao (Gypsum Fibrosum, raw)
Huanglian (Rhizoma Coptidis)
Huangqin (Radix Scutellariae)
Shengdi (Radix Rehmanniae)
Chishao (Radix Paeoniae Rubra)
Dengxin (Medulla Junci)
Qingshu Yiqi Tang (Decoction for Clearing Summer Heat and Tonifying Qi)
Xiyangshen (Western Ginseng)
Maidong (Radix Ophiopogonis)
Zhimu (Rhizoma Anemarrhenae)
Gancao (Radix Glycyrrhizae)
Zhuye (Herba Lophatheri) .
Huanglian (Rhizoma Coptidis)
Shihu (Herba Dendrobii)
Hegeng (Caulis Nelumbinis)
Water melon peel
Rice
Qingwen Baidu Yin (Decoction for Clearing Evil Heat

and Relieving Toxins)
Shigao (Gypsum Fibrosum)
Shengdi (Radix Rehmanniae)
Xijiao (Cornu Rhinoceri Asiatici)
Huanglian (Rhizoma Coptidis)
Zhizi (Fructus Gardeniae)
Jiegeng (Radix Platycodi)
Huangqin (Radix Scutellariae)
Zhimu (Rhizoma Anemarrhenae)
Chishao (Radix Paeoniae Rubra)
Xuanshen (Radix Scrophularia)
Lianqiao (Fructus Forsythiae)
Gancao (Radix Glycyrrhizae)
Danpi (Cortex Moutan Radicis)
Zhuye (Herba Lophatheri)

R

Renshen Wuweizi Tang (Decoction of Radix Ginseng and Fructus Schisandrae)
  Dangshen (Radix Codonopsis Pilosulae)
  Baizhu (Rhizoma Atractylodis Macrocephalae)
  Fuling (Poria)
  Wuweizi (Fructus Schisandrae)
  Maidong (Radix Ophiopogonis)
  Zhigancao (Radix Glycyrrhizae, treated)
  Shengjiang (Rhizoma Zingiberis Recens)
Ruyi Jinhuang San (Golden Yellow Powder for Good Luck)
  Tianhuafen (Radix Trichosanthis)
  Huangbai (Cortex Phellodendri)
  Dahuang (Radix et Rhizoma Rhei)

Baizhi (Radix Angelicae Dahuricae)
Jianghuang (Rhizoma Curcumae Longae)
Shengnanxing (Rhizoma Arisaematis, raw)
Cangzhu (Rhizoma Atractylodis)
Houpo (Cortex Magnoliae Officinalis)
Chenpi (Pericarpium Citri Reticulatae)
Gancao (Radix Glycyrrhizae)

S

Sanao Tang (Decoction of Three Ingredients for Eliminating Wind-cold)
　Mahuang (Herba Ephedrae)
　Xingren (Semen Armeniacae Amarum)
　Gancao (Radix Glycyrrhizae)
Sangbaipi Tang (Decoction of Cortex Mori Radicis)
　Sangbaipi (Cortex Mori Radicis)
　Banxia (Rhizoma Pinelliae)
　Suzi (Fructus Perillae)
　Xingren (Semen Armeniacae Amarum)
　Zhebeimu (Bulbus Fritillariae Thunbergii)
　Huangqin (Radix Scutellariae)
　Huanglian (Rhizoma Coptidis)
　Shanzhi (Fructus Gardeniae)
Sang Ju Yin (Decoction of Folium Mori and Flos Chrysanthemi)
　Sangye (Folium Mori)
　Juhua (Flos Chrysanthemi)
　Xingren (Semen Armeniacae Amarum)
　Lianqiao (Fructus Forsythiae)
　Bohe (Herba Menthae)
　Gancao (Radix Glycyrrhizae)

Jiegeng (Radix Platycodi)

Lugen (Rhizoma Phragmitis)

Sanmiao Wan (Pill of Three Ingredients with Wonderful Effects)

Cangzhu (Rhizoma Atractylodis)

Huangbai (Cortex Phellodendri)

Niuxi (Radix Achyranthis Bidentatae)

Sanzi Yangqin Tang (Decoction of Three Ingredients for Conducting Perverse Qi Downward and Resolving Phlegm-Damp)

Suzi (Fructus Perillae)

Laifuzi (Semen Raphani)

Baijiezi (Semen Sinapis Albae)

Shashen Maidong Tang (Decoction of Radix Glehniae and Radix Ophiopogonis)

Shashen (Radix Glehniae)

Maidong (Radix Ophiopogonis)

Yuzhu (Rhizoma Polygonati Odorati)

Gancao (Radix Glycyrrhizae)

Sangye (Folium Mori)

Baibiandou (Semen Dolichoris Album)

Tianhuafen (Radix Trichosanthis)

Shen Fu Long Mu Jiuni Tang (Decoction of Radix Ginseng, Radix Aconiti Praeparata, Os Draconis and Concha Ostreae for Rescuing the Collapsing State)

Renshen (Radix Ginseng)

Fuzi (Radix Aconiti Praeparata)

Longgu (Os Draconis)

Muli (Concha Ostreae)

Baishao (Radix Paeoniae Alba)

Zhigancao (Radix Glycyrrhizae, treated)

Shen Fu Tang (Decoction of Radix Ginseng and Radix Aconitri Praeparata)

Renshen (Radix Ginseng)

Fuzi (Radix Aconiti Praeparata)

Shen Ling Baizhu San (Powder of Radix Ginseng, Poria and Rhizoma Atractylodis Macrocephalae)

Renshen (Radix Ginseng)

Baizhu (Rhizoma Atractylodis Macrocephalae)

Fuling (Poria)

Gancao (Radix Glycyrrhizae)

Yiren (Semen Coicis)

Jiegeng (Radix Platycodi)

Shanyao (Rhizoma Dioscoreae)

Biandou (Semen Dolichoris Album)

Lianzirou (Semen Neluminis, meat)

Sharen (Fructus Amomi)

Dazao (Fructus Ziziphi Jujubae)

Shenqi San (Powder for Arresting Oozing of Fluid from the Umbilicus)

Kufan (Alum, calcined)

Longgu (Os Draconis)

Shexiang (Moschus)

Shenxian Huoming Yin (Immortal Decoction for Saving Life)

Longdancao (Radix Gentianae)

Xuanshen (Radix Scrophulariae)

Huangbai (Cortex Phellodendri)

Banlangen (Radix Isatidis)

Gualoupi (Fructus Trichosanthis, peel)

Shigao (Gypsum Fibrosum)

Madouling (Fructus Aristolochiae)

Baishao (Radix Paeoniae Alba)

Gancao (Radix Glycyrrhizae)

Shanzhi (Fructus Gardeniae)

Shengdi (Radix Rehmanniae)

Shihu Yeguang Wan (Pill of Herba Dendrobii for Night
    Brightness)
    Tiandong (Radix Asparagi)
    Renshen (Radix Ginseng)
    Fuling (Poria)
    Maidong (Radix Ophiopogonis)
    Shudi (Radix Rehmanniae Praeparata)
    Shengdi (Radix Rehmanniae)
    Tusizi (Semen Cuscutae)
    Juhua (Flos Chrysanthemi)
    Caojueming (Semen Cassiae)
    Xingren (Semen Armeniacae Amarum)
    Shanyao (Rhizoma Dioscoreae)
    Gouqizi (Fructus Lycii)
    Niuxi (Radix Achyranthis Bidentatae)
    Wuweizi (Fructus Schisandrae)
    Baijili (Fructus Tribuli)
    Shihu (Herba Dendrobii)
    Roucongrong (Herba Cistanchis)
    Chuanxiong (Rhizoma Ligustici Chuanxiong)
    Zhigancao (Radix Glycyrrhizae, treated)
    Zhiqiao (Fructus Aurantii)
    Qingxiangzi (Semen Celosiae)
    Fangfeng (Radix Ledebouriellae)
    Huanglian (Rhizoma Coptidis)
    Xijiao (Cornu Rhinoceri Asiatici)
    Lingyangjiao (Cornu Antelopis)
    Shijunzi San (Fructus Quisqualis Powder)
    Shijunzi (Fructus Quisqualis)
    Kulianzi (Fructus Meliae)
    Baiwuyi (Fructus Ulmi Macrocarpae)
    Gancao (Radix Glycyrrhizae)
Simiao Wan (Pill of Four Wonderful Ingredients)

Cangzhu (Rhizoma Atractylodis)
Huangbai (Cortex Phellodendri)
Niuxi (Radix Achyranthis Bidentatae)
Yiren (Semen Coicis)
Suoquan Wan (Pill for Reducing Urine)
Shanyao (Rhizoma Dioscoreae)
Wuyao (Radix Linderae)
Yizhiren (Fructus Alpiniae Oxyphyllae)

T

Tingli Dazao Xiefei Tang (Decoction of Semen Lepidii-
seu Descurainiae and Fructus Ziziphi Jujubae for
Reducing the Lung)
Tinglizi (Semen Lepidii seu Descurainiae)
Dazao (Fructus Ziziphi Jujubae)
Wenxia Qingshang Tang (Decoction for Warming the
Bottom and Clearing Heat on the Top)
Fuzi (Radix Aconiti Praeparata)
Huanglian (Rhizoma Coptidis)
Cishi (Magnetitum)
Gefen (Concha Meretricis seu Cyclinae)
Tianhuafen (Radix Trichosanthis)
Buguzhi (Fructus Psoraleae)
Fupenzi (Fructus Rubi)
Tusizi (Semen Cuscutae)
Sangpiaoxiao (Ootheca Mantidis)
Bailianxu (Stamen Nelumbinis)
Wuling San (Poria Powder in Five Ingredients)
Baizhu (Rhizoma Atractylodis Macrocephalae)
Guizhi (Ramulus Cinnamomi)
Zhuling (Polyporus Umbellatus)

Zexie (Rhizoma Alismatis)
Fuling (Poria)
Wumei Wan (Fructus Mume Pill)
Wumei (Fructus Mume)
Xixin (Herba Asari)
Ganjiang (Rhizoma Zingiberis)
Huanglian (Rhizoma Coptidis)
Danggui (Radix Angelicae Sinensis)
Fuzi (Radix Aconiti Praeparata)
Huangbai (Cortex Phellodendri)
Guizhi (Ramulus Cinnamomi)
Renshen (Radix Ginseng)
Chuanjiao (Pericarpium Zanthoxyli)
Wuwei Xiaodu Yin (Decoction of Five Ingredients for
    Relieving Toxins)
Yinhua (Flos Lonicerae)
Juhua (Flos Chrysanthemi)
Pugongying (Herba Taraxaci)
Zihuadiding (Herba Violae)
Qingtiankui (Herba Semiaquilegiae)
Xiang Sha Liujunzi Wan (Pill of Six Noble Ingredients
    plus Radix Aucklandiae and Fructus Amomi)
Renshen (Radix Ginseng)
Baizhu (Rhizoma Atractylodis Macrocephalae)
Fuling (Poria)
Gancao (Radix Glycyrrhizae)
Banxia (Rhizome Pinelliae)
Chenpi (Pericarpium Citri Reticulatae)
Muxiang (Radix Aucklandiae)
Sharen (Fructus Amomi)
Shengjiang (Rhizoma Zingiberis Recens)
Dazao (Fructus Ziziphi Jujubae)
Xiaoer Huichun Dan (Regeneration Pill for Children)

Niuhuang (Calculus Bovis)
Bingpian (Borneolum Syntheticum)
Zhusha (Cinnabaris)
Qianghuo (Rhizoma seu Radix Notopterygii)
Jiangcan (Bombyx Batryticatus)
Tianma (Rhizoma Gastrodiae)
Fangfeng (Radix Ledebouriellae)
Shexiang (Moschus)
Xionghuang (Realgar)
Dannanxing (Arisaema cum Bile)
Tianzhuhuang (Bamboo Fungus)
Chuanbeimu (Bulbus Fritillariae Cirrhosae)
Quanxi (Scorpio)
Fuzi (Radix Aconiti Praeparata)
Shehanshi (Biferric Trioxide)
Gancao (Radix Glycyrrhizae)
Gouteng (Ramulus Uncariae cum Uncis)
Xiaoqinglong Tang (Decoction of Minor Green Dragon)
Mahuang (Herba Ephedrae)
Guizhi (Ramulus Cinnamomi)
Xingren (Semen Armeniacae Amarum)
Zhigancao (Radix Glycyrrhizae, treated)
Shengshigao (Gypsum Fibrosum, raw)
Shengjiang (Rhizoma Zingiberis Recens)
Dazao (Fructus Ziziphi Jujubae)
Xijiao Dihuang Tang (Decoction of Cornu Rhinoceri Asiatici and Radix Rehmanniae)
Xijiao (Cornu Rhinoceri Asiatici)
Danpi (Cortex Moutan Radicis)
Shengdi (Radix Rehmanniae)
Baishao (Radix Paeoniae Alba)
Xilei San (Powder for Relieving Throat Erosion)

Bingpian (Borneolum Syntheticum)
Renzhijia (Finger nail of man)
Zhenzhu (Margarita)
Niuhuang (Calculus Bovis)
Xiangyaxie (Ivory bit)
Qingdai (Indigo Naturalis)
Bixicao (Nest of Uroctea Compactilis Koch)
Xingjia Xiangru Yin (Newly Revised Decoction of Herba
Elsholtziae seu Moslae)
Xiangru (Herba Elsholtziae seu Moslae)
Yinhua (Flos Lonicerae)
Xianbiandouhua (Flos Dolichoris Album, fresh)
Houpo (Cortex Magnoliae Officinalis)
Lianqiao (Fructus Forsythiae)
Xing Su San (Powder of Semen Armeniacae Amarum
and Folium Perillae)
Xingren (Semen Armeniacae Amarum)
Suye (Folium Perillae)
Juhong (Exocarpium Citri Gradis)
Banxia (Rhizoma Pinelliae)
Jiegeng (Radix Platycodi)
Zhiqiao (Fructus Aurantii)
Qianhu (Radix Peucedani)
Fuling (Poria)
Gancao (Radix Glycyrrhizae)
Dazao (Fructus Ziziphi Jujubae)
Shengjiang (Rhizoma Zingiberis Recens)

Y

Yangyin Qingfei Tang (Decoction for Nourishing Yin
and Clearing Heat in the Lung)

Shengdi (Radix Rehmanniae)
Maidong (Radix Ophiopogonis)
Xuanshen (Radix Scrophulariae)
Danpi (Cortex Moutan Radicis)
Chishao (Radix Paeoniae Rubra)
Zhebeimu (Bulbus Fritillariae Thunbergii)
Gancao (Radix Glycyrrhizae)
Bohe (Herba Menthae)
Yangyin Shengji San (Powder for Nourishing Yin and Producing Muscles)
Shigao (Gypsum Fibrosum)
Xionghuang (Realgar)
Huangbai (Cortex Phellodendri)
Longdancao (Radix Gentianae)
Puhuang (Pollen Typhae)
Qingdai (Indigo Naturalis)
Bohe (Herba Menthae)
Ercha (Ramulus Acaciae)
Gancao (Radix Glycyrrhizae)
Bingpian (Borneolum Syntheticum)
Yinchenhao Tang (Decoction of Herba Artemisiae Scopariae)
Yinchen (Herba Artemisiae Scopariae)
Zhizi (Fructus Gardeniae)
Dahuang (Radix et Rhizoma Rhei)
Yinchen Lizhong Tang (Decoction of Herba Artemisiae Scopariae for Regulating the Middle Jiao)
Yinchen (Herba Artemisiae Scopariae)
Dangshen (Radix Codonopsis Pilosulae)
Ganjiang (Rhizoma Zingiberis)
Baizhu (Rhizoma Atractylodis Macrocephalae)
Gancao (Radix Glycyrrhizae)
Yinqiao San (Powder of Flos Lonicerae and Fructus

Forsythiae)
Yinhua (Flos Lonicerae)
Lianqiao (Fructus Forsythiae)
Douchi (Semen Sojae Praeparatum)
Niubangzi (Fructus Arctii)
Jingjie (Herba Schizonepetae)
Bohe (Herba Menthae)
Jiegeng (Radix Platycodi)
Gancao (Radix Glycyrrhizae)
Zhuye (Herba Lophatheri)
Lugen (Rhizoma Phragmitis)
Yupingfeng San (Jade Screen Powder)
Huangqi (Radix Astragali)
Baizhu (Rhizoma Atractylodis Macrocephalae)
Fangfeng (Radix Ledebouriellae)
Yushu Dan (Jade Pivot Pill)
Shancigu (Rhizoma Pleionis)
Shexiang (Moschus)
Qianjinzishuang (Semen Euphorbiae Degelarinatum)
Xionghuang (Realgar)
Hongyadaji (Radix Knoxiae)
Zhusha (Cinnabaris)
Wubeizi (Galla Chinensis)

Z

Zengye Tang (Decoction for Producing Fluid)
Xuanshen (Radix Scrophlariae)
Maidong (Radix Ophiopogonis)
Xishengdi (Radix Rehmanniae)
Zhenwu Tang (Decoction for Warming the Kidney)
Paofuzi (Radix Aconiti Praeparata)

Baizhu (Rhizoma Atractylodis Macrocephalae)
Fuling (Poria)
Baishao (Radix Paeoniae Alba)
Shengjiang (Rhizoma Zingiberis Recens)
Zhijing San (Powder for Relieving Convulsion)
Quanxie (Scorpio)
Wugong (Scolopendra)
Tianma (Rhizoma Gastrodiae)
Jiangcan (Bombyx Batryticatus)
Zhuli Datan Wan (Bamboo Juice Pill for Dispelling Phlegm)
Dahuang (Radix et Rhizoma Rhei)
Huangqin (Radix Scutellariae)
Banxia (Rhizoma Pinelliae)
Juhong (Exocarpium Citri Grandis)
Jinmengshi (Mica-schist)
Chenxiang (Lignum Aquilariae Resinatum)
Gancao (Radix Glycyrrhizae)
Zhuli (Bamboo juice obtained with heating)
Jiangzhi (ginger juice)